Accession no.

✔ KU-743-289

Writing for Nursing and Midwifery Students

JET LIBRARY

www.thestudyspace.com – the leading study skills website

Study Skills

Academic Success
Academic Writing Skills for International Students
The Business Student's Phrase Book
Cite Them Right (10th edn)
Critical Thinking and Persuasive Writing for
  Postgraduates
The Employability Journal
Essentials of Essay Writing
Get Sorted
Great Ways to Learn Anatomy and Physiology
  (2nd edn)
How to Begin Studying English Literature (4th edn)
How to Use Your Reading in Your Essays (3rd edn)
How to Write Better Essays (4th edn)
How to Write Your Undergraduate Dissertation
  (2nd edn)
Improve Your Grammar (2nd edn)
The Mature Student's Handbook
Mindfulness for Students
The Palgrave Student Planner
The Personal Tutor's Handbook
Presentation Skills for Students (3rd edn)
The Principles of Writing in Psychology
Professional Writing (3rd edn)
Smart Thinking
Stand Out from the Crowd
The Student Phrase Book
The Student's Guide to Writing (3rd edn)
Studying in English
Studying History (4th edn)
Studying Law (4th edn)
Studying Physics
Study Skills for International Postgraduates
Success in Academic Writing (2nd edn)
The Undergraduate Research Handbook (2nd edn)
The Work-Based Learning Student Handbook
  (2nd edn)
Writing for Engineers (4th edn)
Writing History Essays (2nd edn)
Writing for Law
Writing for Nursing and Midwifery Students
  (3rd edn)
Writing for Science Students
Write it Right (2nd edn)

Pocket Study Skills

14 Days to Exam Success (2nd edn)
Analyzing a Case Study
Blogs, Wikis, Podcasts and More

Brilliant Writing Tips for Students
Completing Your PhD
Doing Research (2nd edn)
Getting Critical (2nd edn)
Managing Stress
Planning Your Dissertation (2nd edn)
Planning Your Essay (2nd edn)
Planning Your PhD
Posters and Presentations
Reading and Making Notes (2nd edn)
Referencing and Understanding Plagiarism
  (2nd edn)
Reflective Writing
Report Writing (2nd edn)
Science Study Skills
Studying with Dyslexia (2nd edn)
Success in Groupwork
Time Management
Where's Your Argument?
Writing for University (2nd edn)

Research Skills

Authoring a PhD
The Foundations of Research (2nd edn)
Getting to Grips with Doctoral Research
Getting Published
The Good Supervisor (2nd edn)
The Lean PhD
PhD by Published Work
The PhD Viva
The PhD Writing Handbook
Planning Your Postgraduate Research
The Postgraduate Research Handbook
  (2nd edn)
The Professional Doctorate
Structuring Your Research Thesis

Career Skills

Excel at Graduate Interviews
The Graduate Career Guidebook
Graduate CVs and Covering Letters
Graduate Entrepreneurship
How to Succeed at Assessment Centres
Social Media for Your Student and Graduate Job
  Search
Work Experience, Placements and Internships

For a complete listing of all our titles in this area please visit
www.macmillanihe.com/study-skills

Writing for Nursing and Midwifery Students

3rd edition

Julio Gimenez

LIS - LIBRARY

Date	Fund SHR
1/2/19	nm-tei
Order No.	
2909315	
University of Chester	

JET LIBRARY

macmillan
international
HIGHER EDUCATION

RED GLOBE
PRESS

© Julio Gimenez, under exclusive licence to Springer Nature Limited 2007, 2011, 2019

All rights reserved. No reproduction, copy or transmission of this publication may be made without written permission.

No portion of this publication may be reproduced, copied or transmitted save with written permission or in accordance with the provisions of the Copyright, Designs and Patents Act 1988, or under the terms of any licence permitting limited copying issued by the Copyright Licensing Agency, Saffron House, 6–10 Kirby Street, London EC1N 8TS.

Any person who does any unauthorized act in relation to this publication may be liable to criminal prosecution and civil claims for damages.

The author has asserted his right to be identified as the author of this work in accordance with the Copyright, Designs and Patents Act 1988.

First edition 2007
Second edition 2011
This edition published 2019 by
RED GLOBE PRESS

Previous editions published by Palgrave

Red Globe Press in the UK is an imprint of Springer Nature Limited, registered in England, company number 785998, of 4 Crinan Street, London, N1 9XW.

Red Globe Press® is a registered trademark in the United States, the United Kingdom, Europe and other countries.

ISBN 978–1–137–53118–6 paperback

This book is printed on paper suitable for recycling and made from fully managed and sustained forest sources. Logging, pulping and manufacturing processes are expected to conform to the environmental regulations of the country of origin.

A catalogue record for this book is available from the British Library.

A catalog record for this book is available from the Library of Congress.

Contents

List of Tables

List of Figures

Acknowledgements

My first debt of gratitude is to those who wrote about *writing* before me and have therefore influenced my views and approach to teaching how to write in specific genres: John Swales, Charles Bazerman, Carolyn R. Miller, Chris Candlin, V. K. Bhatia and Ken Hyland, among many others.

I am also indebted to Suzannah Burywood, my commissioning editor, for her support and encouragement. I would also like to thank the four reviewers of the book whose comments have made this a better project. I did not always follow their advice, however, so the remaining flaws are my entire responsibility.

I am thankful to my colleagues at Middlesex University who provided me with enlightening comments during the writing process. Special thanks go to Victoria Odeniyi and Gillian Lazar at ELLS. I am similarly grateful to Clare Maher and Jane Raymond for their invaluable comments and support with the discipline-specific contents of the book, and to Dilys Hall for introducing me to RefWorks. I am equally thankful to my colleague and friend Beverly Fairfax for her comments and feedback on the first draft of the book.

This new edition has benefited immensely from the comments made by a large number of nursing, midwifery and writing lecturers who have adopted the book, and the many students who have also provided me with invaluable feedback. To all of them, I remain indebted.

I am thankful to EndNote and RefWorks for permission to reproduce the screenshots on pages 176–179, and Refbase for permission to reproduce a screenshot of their main page on page 180.

To my students past and present who have given me the best a teacher can get, challenging comments and questions, thank you. Most of the ideas and materials in this book started as answers to such comments and questions.

These acknowledgements would be incomplete without thanking my family and colleagues who have once more believed in my projects; all my gratitude for their love and patience.

Julio Gimenez
University of Westminster, London, UK

Introduction

One of the most difficult tasks we are faced with when we enter university is *writing*. Not only are we asked to deal with new content, we are also required to engage in new intellectual processes and, in many cases, we must even learn to organize and structure knowledge in new ways. Writing, and especially writing assignments, becomes even more taxing for adult students who have been away from formal education for quite some time and come back to university via top-up courses or 'back-to-practice' programmes.

This book has been designed and organized to help you with your writing tasks throughout your undergraduate programme. It combines the theoretical approach of a textbook with the practical activities of a workbook.

Starting with the basic principles of writing at university level, the book first explores the academic essay, then analyses typical genres such as the care critique and the article review, and finally deals with argumentative writing and preparation for the undergraduate dissertation. It includes authentic essay questions and examples at different levels of writing, along with exercises on how to write more effective nursing and midwifery texts.

The book also includes:

- An examination of different **referencing systems** such as the Harvard and the American Psychological Association (APA) styles.
- An introduction to the most common **bibliographical software** used at universities.
- A **glossary of key terms** that expands on the core concepts presented in the 'glossary boxes' in the book and that provides further examples.
- A list of **further readings and resources** that includes links to web-based materials.
- **Suggested answers** to activities, which will be very useful if you are working on your own.
- An **achievement chart** to help you keep a record of your progress.

What makes this book different

You will also find that the book is:

- **Specific** – it has been designed to meet the specific writing needs of student nurses and midwives. The book deals with the writing genres you will be asked to produce, from the academic and the reflective essay and the care critique to research proposals, reports and the dissertation.
- **Easy to use** – you will find that the 'how to' chapters cover all the main writing genres in a practical, step-by-step way.
- **Active and engaging** – the chapters have been written in a very engaging style. Reading them will not be a solitary activity; you will find a tutor every step of the way.
- **Comprehensive** – in addition to the main writing genres, you will find chapters on how to avoid plagiarism, how to use web-based bibliography managers, sample essay questions and how to answer them to meet typical marking criteria, and advice on grammar and language for the ESOL student.
- **Up to date** – the content is based on current theory and practice in nursing and midwifery and is aligned with the general benchmark statements of international quality assurance associations.

I hope that by the end of the book you will feel more confident about writing in general, and writing in the specific genres of nursing and midwifery in particular. Like any other type of writing, academic writing is a purposeful activity whose main aim is to satisfy the needs of its readers. And this is what I *really* hope this book will achieve.

The third edition

The third edition of *Writing for Nursing and Midwifery Students* has been revised and augmented to include:

- A number of writing genres (e.g. case studies, systematic reviews) which in the past few years have become more central to nursing and midwifery.
- An extended section on argumentative writing.
- An extended section on writing research proposals.
- A more detailed section on reporting verbs used in paraphrasing and quoting other people's texts.
- An updated section on reference management software.
- An enlarged glossary.
- An improved index.

The Essentials of Academic Writing

The chapters in this part introduce you to the basics of writing in an academic environment, with a focus on your specific needs as a student of nursing or midwifery. First, you will explore the principles of organizing and structuring information and see how these principles work for different kinds (and levels) of nursing and midwifery writing. You will then look at description and argumentation and see how these can be put to work in different writing genres. Finally, you will examine more complex processes such as reflection and critical thinking.

CHAPTER 1: AN INTRODUCTION TO ACADEMIC WRITING

In this first chapter, you will find the essentials of academic writing at university level. The chapter starts by exploring background (what), rationale (why) and signposting (how) in essay planning. It then introduces the principles of 'macro structuring'. It will show you how to expand the structure of a paragraph into an essay, organize information in order to enhance the flow of your texts and structure ideas following an organizing principle. Next, the chapter considers 'micro structuring' at the paragraph level. At the end of the chapter, you will find suggestions for dealing with common grammar and English use problems, such as sentence fragments, incorrect punctuation and dangling modifiers.

CHAPTER 2: EXPLORING ACADEMIC GENRES

Chapter 2 elaborates on the principles explored in the first chapter. It illustrates how these principles work for the typical texts or genres you will be asked to produce at the different levels of your undergraduate studies. In line with the demands of most university courses, the chapter works from description to argumentation. It thus starts with the generic academic essay and moves on to explore more specific genres, such as the care critique and the article review. In the last part of the chapter, you will examine argumentation for the argumentative essay.

CHAPTER 3: PROCESSES IN ACADEMIC WRITING

This chapter will help you explore two complex processes that have a direct bearing on writing: reflection and critical thinking. You will start by looking at what reflection involves and at how the different stages of the reflection cycle can be incorporated into the reflective essay. The chapter then introduces you to the principles of critical thinking and how you can use these principles to evaluate your sources of reference.

An Introduction to Academic Writing

At the end of this chapter, you should be able to:

- recognize the five basic principles of planning in academic writing
- identify the three elements in essay questions and follow marking criteria
- understand gathering, organizing and structuring information
- reproduce the generic structure of academic texts
- identify main problems with sentence fragments, cohesion, dangling modifiers and punctuation.

The basics of planning in academic writing

Have you ever written a letter? An email? Even a short mobile text? If you have, you wrote for a purpose. It was a **purposeful activity**. Academic writing is also a purposeful activity. When you write an assignment, you have a definite purpose in mind. You want a particular audience (who?) to have information (what?) with a specific focus (what exactly?). You have reasons for doing so (why?), and you are delivering the information in a certain way, such as describing, discussing or analysing (how?).

These five question words (*who, what, what exactly, why* and *how*) can be your **guiding prompts** when you plan your next piece of writing.

Let us look at an example. Suppose you had to write an essay on the following: *Midwife means 'with woman'. Discuss how the midwife should care for the woman in the second stage of labour.* You could use the five question words above to ask yourself some guiding questions. For instance:

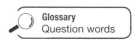
Glossary
Question words

Audience:	**Who** am I writing the essay for? *Lecturer.*
Topic:	**What** is the essay going to be about? *Midwife care for the woman in labour.*
Focus:	**What exactly** am I going to focus on? *Some ways in which the midwife can provide care in the second stage of labour.*

Rationale: **Why** am I going to focus on some ways of providing care and not others? *They are the most crucial at this stage of labour.*

Signpost: **How** am I going to deliver the information? *By discussing the different ways the midwife can provide the care.*

These questions will help you choose the right information for your essay as well as the right amount of information for your audience. Your course lecturer, your audience in this case, already knows the answer to the essay question and probably expects you to answer it in a certain way. But your lecturer does not exactly know what information you will choose or why you will choose it. This is the **rationale** for your essay. It is what makes your essay unique – only you will choose to deal with the topic in the way you have decided.

These questions give you the five basic principles of essay planning. They will help you organize your ideas and structure your information so that your essay has the focus you want it to have. Organizing and structuring your information in this way will also improve the flow of your texts. You will need more information to develop your essay, but the five questions give you the basic approach to planning any academic text. When your lecturer finishes reading your assignment, s/he should know why you have answered the essay question in the way you have.

Glossary
Rationale
Signpost

Planning and structuring principles

One possible way of planning your essays is by following the five basic questions that represent basic **planning and structuring principles**. Figure 1.1 shows how you can go about planning to answer an essay question.

Figure 1.1 illustrates how you can organize your essay (for example from general to specific) and how you can structure it (from background information to examples). When you decide to arrange the information in your text from general

General

TOPIC (what) / **AUDIENCE** (for whom)

FOCUS (what exactly) / **RATIONALE** (why)

SIGNPOST (how)

SUPPORTING EVIDENCE / EXAMPLES

Specific

Figure 1.1 **Planning essays**

to specific, as in this case, or from most to least important or chronologically (from most recent to oldest), you are using an **organizing principle**. But when you decide that your text will present your reader with some background information before the focus and the rationale, as shown in Figure 1.1, you are planning the **structuring principle** for your text.

Remember that whereas organization can easily be changed, structure is not as flexible. Structure is connected with the way we transmit and understand new and given information. Structuring tends to be fairly fixed, and it largely depends on the language we are using. In English writing, background information normally precedes supporting examples. It is always a good idea to choose your organizing principle first and then decide on the most appropriate structure for your information.

You may decide, for example, that the information in your essay will be organized from general to specific. Then you may choose to structure it giving the background information first, and then the examples. Thus, your text will present:

- **Background information** on the topic (what).
- The **focus** (what exactly).
- The **rationale** for answering the essay question in a particular way (why).
- The **signpost** (how the information will be delivered: by description, analysis, discussion etc.).

Understanding essay questions

You will find many of the ideas we have just discussed in essay questions themselves. Essay questions can tell you what information to include (what), what aspects of that information to include (what exactly) and how you should deliver such aspects (how). If you analyse essay questions carefully, you will discover that most contain these three basic elements: the **topic**, the **focus** and the **signpost**. How you approach the topic is entirely up to you and, as we said, that is what makes your essay different from all other essays.

Let us consider again the essay question:

Midwife means 'with woman'. Discuss how the midwife should care for the woman in the second stage of labour.

The topic is the care that the midwife should provide for the woman. This is very broad and you could include many things in your discussion. You could, for example, think of prenatal and postnatal care, health promotion and care that meets the woman's social needs. However, the essay question asks about *the second stage of labour*. Many of these aspects of midwifery care are only *indirectly* connected to the second stage of labour, which is the aspect on which you need to focus your writing. Therefore, you need to narrow down your focus. You should then consider aspects like:

- How does the midwife's role change in the second stage?
- How do the woman's needs change in the second stage?
- This stage is called the 'pushing stage' – what is actually happening?
- Should the midwife go for 'spontaneous pushing' or 'sustained directed bearing-down efforts'?
- How can the midwife support the woman emotionally until the baby is born?

Narrowing down will help you stay focused and avoid including information that is not relevant to the topic. Finally, you should look at the **verb** to see how your lecturer expects you to develop your answer. The verb in the question will indicate how you need to signpost your essay. What is the verb in the example essay question? Does it ask you to:

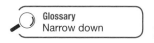

Glossary
Narrow down

- Say what is right or wrong about the care that the midwife should provide in the second stage of labour?
- Examine different aspects of the care in the second stage of labour?

'Discuss' does not mean say what is right or wrong. It means examine different aspects of a topic. You could, for instance, think of the midwife's care in term of physical support (for example suggesting alternative positions for women without epidural anaesthesia, helping with contractions) and of emotional support (for example dealing with intense emotions and sensations). In this way, you could examine the different roles that the midwife could play in the second stage and, using **supporting evidence** from the literature or from your clinical placement (see later in the chapter), discuss alternatives in relation to physical and emotional support. As this example shows, verbs in essay questions are essential for understanding how you are supposed to signpost your essay.

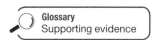

Glossary
Supporting evidence

Let us look at another example. This time we will examine a typical question for nursing students:

Evaluate the importance of effective communication in nursing.

Again, you should identify the topic first: *communication in nursing*. Remember that topics tend to be broad, so you will need a focus. In this example question, the focus is given by the phrase 'the importance of effective communication'. You will need to tell your reader 'what effective communication in nursing' is and 'why it is important'.

You could, for example, include ideas such as 'communication with other nurses, clients and the client's family', 'what makes each type of communication effective' and 'the importance of verbal communication on admission to hospital'.

The table below lists the verbs you will see most often used in essay questions. Write the meaning of each verb in your own words. You do not need to provide complete sentences; key words will do. Use a dictionary if you are not sure of the meanings. 'Argue' and 'discuss' have been completed for you as examples.

Verb	Definition	Additional information
Analyse		
Argue	To give reasons why something is right or wrong, true or untrue.	To persuade people.
Classify		
Demonstrate		
Differentiate		
Discuss	To examine in detail, showing the different opinions or ideas about something.	Frequently confused with 'argue', but a more balanced response is required in 'discuss'.
Evaluate		
Examine		
Explain		
Identify		
Outline		
Produce		

Answers *See suggested answers on p. 192.*

Finally, you need to consider the signpost; that is, the action you are asked to take in relation to the topic and its focus. In this example, the action is 'evaluate', so you are to judge the value of effective communication in nursing to form an opinion about it (see Activity 1.1 above and the suggested answers to it at the back of the book).

Interpreting and using marking criteria

As well as the essay question, you should also look at the **marking criteria** for the essay. These criteria are an important source of information for you. They will help you make decisions on what to include in your essay. Using the marking criteria at the planning stage will improve your chances of getting a higher mark.

Glossary
Assessment/marking criteria

Table 1.1 Sample marking criteria for a short essay	
Criteria	Comments
1. Work neatly presented and easy to read	
2. Evidence of self-assessment of skills at the beginning of the semester	
3. Balanced view of the progress made in each of the skills	
4. Identification of further developmental needs	
5. Correct spelling and grammar	
6. List of references included	

Here is another example. This is a question for a 1000-word reflective essay and Table 1.1 gives its accompanying marking criteria:

Discuss how your transferable skills of communication, effective learning, teamwork, numeracy, and personal and career development have developed during the semester.

Did you realize that half the total marking criteria for this assignment are for the conventions of academic writing? Let us examine each of these three criteria in more detail.

Criterion 1 refers to the presentation of your work and how easy it is to read. A well-presented essay may get a higher mark than a disorganized and poorly presented one. Here are some important things to keep in mind. Your essay should be:

- Word processed, with no typing errors.
- Double spaced throughout.
- Written in a legible **font style** and **font size** – normally using Times New Roman or Arial, 11 or 12 pt.
- Presented with generous margins – generally 2 to 2.5 centimetres all round.
- Correctly introduced (see the section on paragraphing below).

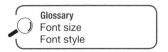

Glossary
Font size
Font style

- Adequately paragraphed (see the section on paragraphing below).

Criterion 5 is also connected with how easy your essay is to read. If the spelling and grammar are correct, you will improve your chances of getting a better mark. You should:

- Use the word processor spell-check, though it is always safer to consult a dictionary as well.

- Refer to a grammar guide if you are unsure of the correct use of the language (see the section on grammar and English use below, and Further Readings and Resources at the end of the book).

Criterion 6 is about referencing, which is discussed in detail in Chapter 10. Here are some basic considerations connected with references. When you prepare your **list of references**, you have to remember to:

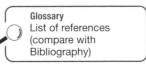

Glossary
List of references
(compare with
Bibliography)

- Include only those references you have mentioned in the body of your text.
- Organize the list of references alphabetically.
- Include the basic information about the references.
- Make sure that there is no discrepancy between the references on the list and those in the text.

Now that you have

- examined the essay question and
- analysed the marking criteria,

you are ready to start the final stage in planning: gathering the information that you will include in your essay.

Gathering information

The final stage in planning is known as 'search and select'. This simply means that you collect as much information about the topic as possible, then choose the most useful. These two processes are closely linked, and are important for organizing and structuring information before you start writing your essay. Figure 1.2 illustrates the links between them.

Searching for information

Where can you start searching for information? Class handouts and class notes can provide excellent starting points. They may contain references that have been suggested by your lecturers, normally in a recommended reading list. These sources of 'pre-selected information' can help you reduce the anxiety created by having to look at too many sources.

The internet is another source of information. But it can also be a source of confusion. When you do an internet search, remember to use key words instead of phrases. For instance, if you wanted to do a search for:

Midwife means 'with woman'. Discuss how the midwife should care for the woman in the second stage of labour

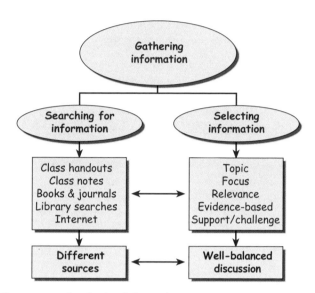

Figure 1.2 **The process of gathering information**

you would be better off using words/phrases like 'second stage' or 'stages of labour'. This will reduce the number of hits you get back as a response to your search. Alternatively, if you want to search for the whole phrase 'the second stage of labour', use inverted commas at the beginning and end of the phrase so as to avoid hitting pages containing meaningless words such as 'the' and 'of'.

A second word of warning about the internet relates to the quality of information you may find. Unlike other sources (such as journals and books), the contents of websites may not be safeguarded for their accuracy and correctness. There are no 'editorial boards' to make sure that what gets published is accurate and correct. Always check for things such as:

- Who is responsible for the website.
- Whether the website is associated with or recognized by a council.
- The academic credentials of the person writing the information.
- The type of audience for which the website was designed.

Once you have established a relationship of trust with a given website, then you can use its information safely.

A more reliable source of information for your academic activities is databases. Access to online databases will be provided by your university library. Academic databases may contain information about books, journals, newspapers, reports and so on. You have to keep in mind that each source is different in its scope and features, so it is always a good idea to start by becoming familiar with the source you will be using. The two main ways to search databases are by using subject headings, also called 'descriptors', and key words. You can get more detailed information on how to make the most of the databases available at your university by using the 'Help' function in the database or by asking a librarian at your university library.

Selecting information

Not all the sources of information you have chosen will find a home in your essay. You will still have to **select** the most appropriate pieces. As shown in Figure 1.2, there are various principles you can follow. You can select information by:

- Its topic.
- Its focus.
- How closely connected it is to your focus.
- Its quality.
- Whether it is evidence-based.

It is also important that you present your reader with an objective and balanced account. For this, you will need to include not only those sources of information that confirm your position but also those that challenge it. We will return to this point when we deal with argumentation in Chapter 2 and, especially, in Chapter 6.

If you manage to strike a balance between books, journal articles and internet content, you will provide your readers with **different sources** of good-quality and updated information. Lecturers will want to see this in your assignments.

If you manage to consider not only relevant and evidence-based materials that support the points you want to make but also those that challenge your arguments, you will provide your audience with a **well-balanced discussion**. Lecturers will want to see this in your assignments too!

> **Glossary**
> Evidence-based

Organizing and structuring information

Now it is time to decide how you will **organize and structure** your essay. Remember that organizing and structuring are two related but slightly different processes. Organization has to do with order, while structuring refers to patterns. If you were working on the different ways in which the midwife can support the woman in the second stage of labour, how could you organize these ways?

One method is by listing. When you list aspects, or ways as in this case, you isolate them and thus you can identify them more clearly. There is also an element of 'classifying' here. Classifying helps with logical thinking, achieving balance and clearer writing. Do not worry about the order of the elements in your list; you can change the order later on. Use bullets rather than numbers so that you do not get any particular order fixed in your head at this stage.

For example, you can list the ways in which the midwife can support the woman physically and emotionally:

Supporting women in the second stage of labour	
A. Physical support	B. Emotional support
Monitor the foetal heart	Talk her through the process
Assess and protect the perineum	Encourage her verbally
Provide equipment, e.g. beanbag	Support choice of position

The next step is to give the selected items a certain order. This step should always be guided by some principle. As we discussed above, you can organize them chronologically, in order of importance, or by dealing with the most difficult first. In this case, we will organize the items following a chronological order:

Supporting women in the second stage of labour	
1. Physical support	2. Emotional support
1.1 Monitor the foetal heart	2.1 Support choice of position
1.2 Provide equipment, e.g. beanbag	2.2 Encourage her verbally
1.3 Assess and protect the perineum	2.3 Talk her through the process

ACTIVITY 1.2

Here are some scrambled ideas about the second essay question we considered above: *Evaluate the importance of effective communication in nursing.* How would you organize and structure them to write an essay on this question? You may need to leave some out, depending on the rationale you have chosen.

The importance of effective communication in nursing

- Collaboration and negotiation skills with clients and families
- Common barriers to effective communication
- Communication as a therapeutic space
- Communicating with the family
- Work teams in nursing practice

- Dealing with aggression
- Focusing on feelings, being warm and non-judgemental
- Self-disclosure and small groups
- Facilitating empathy

Answers See suggested answers on p. 193.

Notice that you can now change bullets into numbers, as this is the order in which the essay will be developed.

Organizing and structuring will help the ideas in your **text flow** more smoothly, while enhancing your chances of a higher mark.

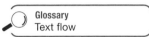

Glossary
Text flow

Paragraphing information

Now that you have finished planning, it is time to shape your information into texts. This process is called **paragraphing**. Paragraphing refers to putting information into 'blocks' or paragraphs that contain one principal idea.

ACTIVITY 1.3

Read the following paragraph and answer the questions below.

Nurses can work in many health-care settings, which gives them the opportunity to gain experience in all aspects of caring for clients and their families. Nurses can thus build their professional career in many different ways. They may choose to become clinical specialists or consultant nurses, or they can opt for managerial positions as a head of nursing services or supervisor of other nurses. Some may prefer to pursue an academic career in education and research. These are just a few examples of the opportunities that nurses currently have to develop their professional interests.

The paragraph has five sentences. Can you identify

1. The sentence that introduces the general idea of the text (**topic**)?
2. Another sentence that provides the focus/point of view of the topic (**focus**)?
3. The examples that develop/support the focus (**examples/evidence**)?
4. The sentence that brings the text to an end (**conclusion**)?

Answers See suggested answers on p. 193.

The first sentence in a paragraph sets the scene for the reader. It discloses the **topic** of the text; that is why it is usually called the 'topic sentence'. This sentence provides the reader with enough background information to understand the text.

The topic and the focus in the paragraph in Activity 1.3 tell us that nurses can build a professional career in many different ways. But which are these ways? To answer this question, we need to go on reading and find either **examples** or **evidence** to support the claims made in the focus. The text in Activity 1.3 uses examples to do this. After the text presents examples exploring different possibilities for nurses, it moves on to a conclusion. The **conclusion**, the fifth sentence in the activity paragraph, brings a text to an end in a satisfactory manner.

But what is a *satisfactory manner*? The answer is in the focus of your text. When you present your readers with the focus of your text, you create certain expectations in them. For example, if you said that you would discuss 'the three fundamental reasons that make the third stage of labour the most critical', your reader would immediately expect to read three fundamental reasons why you consider the third stage of labour the most critical.

A satisfactory conclusion also takes the reader back to the focus of the text. In the text about careers for nurses, we can clearly see how the conclusion **rephrases** (states the same idea by using similar words) the focus of the text. Thus, we can draw a parallel between the focus of the text ('nurses can thus build their professional career in many different ways') and its conclusion ('these are just a few examples of the opportunities that nurses currently have to develop their professional interests'). This conclusion is also satisfactory because it gives the reader something further to think about. The writer is inviting the reader to 'engage' with the ideas in the text by thinking of other ways in which nurses can develop their careers or professional interests. Good conclusions always leave the reader with something to think about.

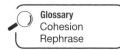

Glossary
Cohesion
Rephrase

There is one last thing we need to consider: how all these parts of the text have been put together. This is called **cohesion**. Cohesion is the 'glue' that sticks the text together. You can create cohesion by:

- Repeating key words that remind the reader of what the text is about and link the ideas expressed in different sentences.
- Using a network of words (e.g. nurses, nursing, care, clients etc.) that helps the writer put ideas together while avoiding heavy repetition of the same word or words.
- Using connectives (e.g. and, but, thus) that give unity to the text and show the connection between one idea and the next, one sentence and the next or even one text and the next (see the section on grammar and English use below).

From paragraph to essay

The basic structure we have just analysed is sometimes referred to as the **generic structure** of a paragraph. A generic structure is like the 'backbone' of a text that can be used to generate similar texts. You can use this generic structure again and again every time you need to create a new paragraph.

The generic structure of a paragraph can be expanded to create the generic structure of an essay, and Figure 1.3 shows how the generic structure of a short text like the paragraph about careers for nurses can be expanded to create the structure of an essay.

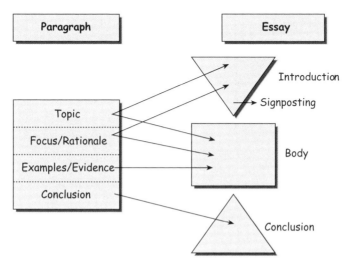

Figure 1.3 **Expanding a paragraph into an essay**
Inspired by Oshima & Hogue (1998) and Swales & Feak (1994).

The inverted triangle in the essay introduction represents the general-to-specific way in which information has been organized. In the conclusion, in contrast, information has been organized from specific to general. We will come back to this at the end of this section.

The function of each part of a paragraph (for example the topic sentence provides the reader with background information about the text) can be mirrored in the function of each part of an essay. So the introduction of an essay will first present the topic, then the focus and then the rationale. The only function that we do not frequently find in a paragraph but that should be present in the introduction of an essay is signposting (how you will deliver the information in your essay).

Figure 1.4 shows how the topic and the focus in the paragraph about careers for nurses can be expanded into the introduction of a short essay.

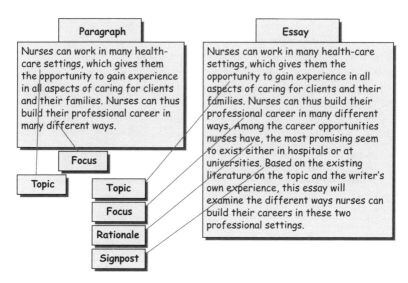

Figure 1.4 From paragraph to essay – example 1

The examples used to support the claims we have made in the focus of the paragraph and in the essay introduction can be organized in different paragraphs in the body of the essay. Figure 1.5 illustrates one way of doing this.

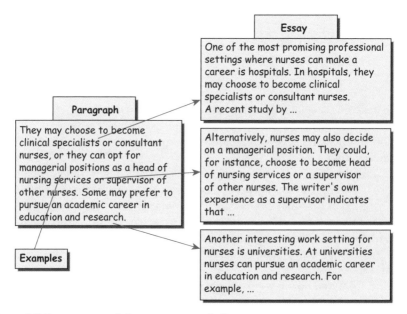

Figure 1.5 From paragraph to essay – example 2

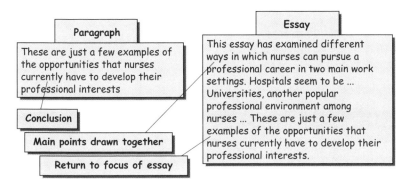

Figure 1.6 **From paragraph to essay – example 3**

Notice how each supporting example has generated one body paragraph in the essay. Can you also see how each of the paragraphs in the body of the essay follows the generic structure we discussed above: topic, focus and evidence or examples to support the claims? Figure 1.6 now shows how the conclusion in the paragraph about careers for nurses can be expanded into the concluding paragraph of the essay.

As you can see, the concluding paragraph in the essay first draws together the main points mentioned in the body of the text by summarizing them. It then returns to the focus of the essay. Notice also that while the information in the introductory paragraph is organized from general to specific, the organization of the information in the conclusion goes from specific to general. Although you may come across variations of this kind of essay organization and structuring, this is a typical ordering and patterning of information in an academic essay.

You will find more on planning, organizing and structuring specific assignments (for example the reflective essay and the care critique) in Part Two of this book.

Grammar and English use

This last section of the chapter deals with some of the main grammar and language-use problems that many students experience when writing academically. We look at sentence fragments, cohesion, dangling modifiers and punctuation. If you feel that you need more detail on any of these topics, see the Glossary of Key Terms and the list of Further Readings and Resources at the end of the book.

Sentence fragments

Sentence fragments are incomplete pieces of writing that do not make sense on their own. The most common fragments (see also Table 1.2) are:

- Phrases without a main verb (e.g. *All treatments available at hospitals.*).

- Parts of a longer sentence that have been used independently (e.g. *Because they made the wrong decision.*).
- Phrases with a verb but without a subject (e.g. *In the end decided to go for a Caesarean operation.*).

Table 1.2 Sentence fragments

Problem	Solution
Phrase without a main verb Some more comments about the procedures. (*a phrase*)	**Add a verb** Some more comments were made about the procedures.
Unconnected fragment Patients were asked to sign consent forms. Before the doctors made a final decision. (*a part of the previous sentence*)	**Join the two parts to make one sentence** Patients were asked to sign consent forms before the doctors made a final decision.
Missing subject Through not carefully monitoring the foetus created a risky situation for both the mother and the baby. (*no subject*)	**Add the doer of the action** Through not carefully monitoring the foetus, they created a risky situation for both the mother and the baby.

Cohesion

Cohesion, as we have seen, refers to the use of words or phrases that allow you to put parts of a text together (see Table 1.3). You can provide cohesion by, for example, repeating key words, creating a network of similar words and using connectives (words or phrases that connect, for instance *and, but, so*). Cohesion is important to make sure that the text flows and to link ideas, paragraphs and longer texts.

Table 1.3 Sentence cohesion

Problem	Solution
Group of choppy sentences Nurses can specialize in different areas. They can, for example, choose to do mental health, dual diagnosis. They can also choose neonatal nursing. Nurses can specialize within hospitals. They can work as a school nurse. They can move out into the community.	**Use connectives** Nurses can specialize in different areas. They can, for example, choose to do mental health, dual-diagnosis or neonatal nursing. They can also specialize within hospitals, work as a school nurse or move out into the community.

Problem	Solution
Little cohesion Breastfeeding can help the mother have a faster recovery after childbirth. The hormones that are normally released during nursing help the uterus return to its normal size. It can reduce bleeding. Nursing mothers can lose weight more easily.	**Use a connective** Breastfeeding can help the mother have a faster recovery after childbirth. The hormones that are normally released during nursing help the uterus return to its normal size. It can **also** reduce bleeding. **In addition**, it has been found that nursing mothers can lose weight more easily.
Very little cohesion with the wider text Nurses can work in many health-care settings, which gives them the opportunity to gain experience in all aspects of care. They can thus build their career in many different ways.	**Create a network of words** Nurses can work in many health-care settings, which gives them the opportunity to gain experience in all aspects of care for **clients** and their **families. Nurses** can thus build their **professional** career in many different ways.

Dangling modifiers

A dangling modifier is a word or a phrase that has no clear connection with the rest of the sentence (see Table 1.4). For example:

Having asked all patients for their consent, the survey was carried out.

In this case, 'having asked all patients for their consent' is dangling (loosely or not clearly connected with the part of the sentence that follows). One important

Table 1.4 Dangling modifiers	
Problem	Solution
Dangling modifier Having finished the shift, all uniforms worn on the day were sent to the laundry.	**Change the subject of the sentence** Having finished the shift, **the caretakers** sent all uniforms worn on the day to the laundry. or **Add a subject to the first part** When **the shift** was finished, all uniforms worn on the day were sent to the laundry.
Dangling modifier Without numeracy skills, drugs cannot be administered to patients.	**Change the subject of the sentence** Without numeracy skills, **nurses** cannot administer drugs to patients. or **Add a subject to the first part** If **nurses** do not have numeracy skills, they cannot administer drugs to their patients.

point to remember here is that phrases at the beginning of a sentence do not have a stated subject but take the subject of the part of the sentence that follows, sometimes creating a humorous effect. Consider another example that appeared in an American newspaper article:

> *While driving on Greenwood Avenue yesterday afternoon, a tree began to fall toward Wendy H's car. [As is, this sounds as if the tree was driving!]*

Punctuation

Punctuation is used to signal a pause, emphasis, expansion or clarification. The most frequently used punctuation marks are the *colon, comma, dash, full stop, parentheses, quotation marks* and *semicolon* (see Table 1.5).

Table 1.5 Problems with punctuation	
Problem	Solution
At this hospital, nurses can specialize in one of three areas, mental health, dual-diagnosis or neonatal nursing.	**Use a colon to introduce other related ideas** At this hospital, nurses can specialize in one of three areas: mental health, dual-diagnosis or neonatal nursing. **NB:** if the colon introduces a list of objects, names or phrases, they should be separated by commas. If the colon introduces complete sentences, they should be separated by semicolons (;).
Before they can register with the council nurses have to have the necessary qualifications.	**Add a comma after an introductory sentence** Before they can register with the council, nurses have to have the necessary qualifications.
After finishing their shift all midwives should sign the register.	**Add a comma after an introductory phrase** After finishing their shift, all midwives should sign the register.
The results contradicted previous studies. However replication of this study has been highly recommended.	**Add a comma after an introductory connective** The results contradicted previous studies. However, replication of this study has been highly recommended.
Doctors, nurses and consultants, considered all the possible ways of saving his life.	**Delete the comma that separates the subject (what is being talked about) from the verb** Doctors, nurses and consultants considered all the possible ways of saving his life.
Organization, structuring and paragraphing, such are the qualities of good academic writing.	**Mark off a summarizing statement with a dash** Organization, structuring and paragraphing – such are the qualities of good academic writing.

Problem	Solution
Midwives should provide their clients with all the necessary information for them to make informed decisions	**Finish a complete sentence (not a question or exclamation) with a full stop** Midwives should provide their clients with all the necessary information for them to make informed decisions.
The consultant, who had received more than one prize, someone said more than a dozen, denied the accusation.	**Put extra, non-essential information between parentheses** The consultant, who had received more than one prize (someone said more than a dozen), denied the accusation.
When this happens, health promotion has proven to be the most effective strategy (Stallen 2003).	**Use quotation marks to enclose somebody else's words** When this happens, health promotion 'has proven to be the most effective strategy' (Stallen 2003, p. 345). Also see Chapters 9 and 10.
They tried all possible ways to save his life however, his heart did not restart.	**Use a semicolon before a connective that connects two sentences** They tried all possible ways to save his life; however, his heart did not restart.

Revising the objectives of this chapter

Tick those objectives that you feel you have achieved and review those you have not yet managed to accomplish. Then, complete the **Achievement Chart** at the back of the book.

In this chapter, you have learnt to:

☐ recognize the five basic principles of planning in academic writing

☐ identify the three elements in essay questions and follow marking criteria

☐ understand gathering, organizing and structuring information

☐ reproduce the generic structure of academic texts

☐ identify the main problems with sentence fragments, cohesion, dangling modifiers and punctuation.

Exploring Academic Genres

At the end of this chapter, you should be able to:

- recognize the difference between description and argumentation
- identify the main academic genres in nursing and midwifery
- understand the purpose and the structure of these academic genres
- identify main language items used in descriptive and critical writing.

From description to argumentation

Have you noticed that an ad for a 'room to let', for example, has a different function from a letter to the editor of a newspaper? Compare the two samples in Figure 2.1.

Sir,
I was really surprised to read that the association of clinical diabetologists claims that more consultants are needed to cope with the increasing epidemic when they know too well that most diabetes care lies in the hands of the GP.

What we REALLY need is more staff and facilities to help GP practices manage the increasing number of patients suffering from diabetes.

Have they not heard that many hospital diabetologists insist on keeping diabetes care in the community?

Dr. D. T.
London

— ROOM TO LET —

A double room with a fridge, new double bed, newly furnished, with a three-door wardrobe, drawer unit and bedside table. TV with cable and internet facility ready. Two large windows. 2 minutes from tube station.

Figure 2.1 'Letter to the editor' vs 'room to let'

While the ad for the room describes its size, furniture, location and so on, the letter to the editor presents a particular claim about a topic that has been recently discussed in the newspaper. The ad is descriptive; the letter to the editor is argumentative.

As an undergraduate student of nursing or midwifery, you will be asked to produce both descriptive and argumentative writing. In the first year of your programme, you will be required to write some descriptive essays in which you mostly describe facts, sometimes with a small amount of analysis. This is normally referred to as 'level 1 writing' and is broadly equivalent to Certificate (C) level in the Quality Assurance Agency (QAA) Framework for Higher Education Qualifications in England, Wales and Northern Ireland.

Glossary
Argumentative writing
Article review
Care critique
Critical analysis
Genres

Towards the end of the first year and the beginning of the second, you will need to start developing your higher-level cognitive skills. This is when you start writing in more evaluative **genres** such as the **care critique** and the **article review**. In the final year of your programme, you will have to write **argumentative essays**, showing a **critical analysis** of the issues explored.

This progression from description to argumentation can be charted on a cline. This cline, shown in Figure 2.2, illustrates how description, critical skills and argumentation are combined as you progress on your programme of study.

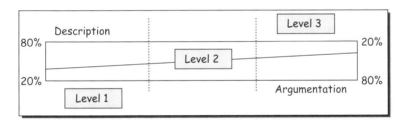

Figure 2.2 The description–argumentation cline

No piece of writing can be 100% descriptive or 100% argumentative. It will always be a combination of the two, but the percentage of each changes as your writing becomes more complex. Figure 2.2 shows how descriptive and argumentative skills combine along the cline. Although there are no hard-and-fast rules for hitting the winning formula, it is fairly common to find an 80–20 combination (80% description and 20% analysis) at the descriptive end of the cline.

Nearing the end of the first year, this combination already starts to change. Around your second year of study, the genres you will be asked to write in require a 40–60 combination, weighting the formula in favour of argumentation. This is called 'writing at level 2' and is roughly equivalent to Intermediate (I) level in the QAA Framework. Towards the completion of your programme, the combination of description and argumentation is completely reversed. At this other end of the cline, you will be producing argumentative essays that require a combination of 20% description and 80% argumentation. This is 'level 3 writing' and should lead to the achievement of some of the Honours (H) level learning outcomes in the QAA Framework.

The genres you will be required to write in can be structurally based on a generic essay, which we call the *academic essay*. This is what we will discuss in the next section.

The academic essay

The academic essay is also known as the three-section essay. It normally has an introductory section, a main body and a concluding section. The way information is organized and structured in this essay is similar to the way the essay about careers for nurses in Chapter 1 was organized.

> **Glossary**
> Generic genre

The academic essay is a **generic genre** that can be used for many purposes. It may:

- Describe facts, issues etc. (the descriptive essay).
- Identify logical relationships (the explanatory essay).
- Compare two or more issues or aspects of a topic (the comparative essay).

It is important to remember that the purpose of your essay should reflect the purpose of the essay question, mainly given by its verb. Is your essay supposed to *describe, explain, compare* or *discuss*? You should also keep in mind that the functions of each section (introduction, body and conclusion) should agree with the general function of your essay. This will enhance the structure and the flow of your text.

In this section of the chapter we will discuss the function of each of the parts of the academic essay, but we will focus mainly on the introduction, as it is here where you signal what the essay will do: describe, explain, identify, compare and so on.

The introduction

One function of the introduction is to tell your reader how you plan to develop your essay (see also Chapter 1). There are several ways in which you may do this, based on what the essay question asks you to do. You may, for example, need to describe facts, identify logical relationships or compare issues relating to a topic.

> **Glossary**
> Logical relationships

It is important that you can identify the connection between your purpose for writing (to answer the question) and the type of essay you need to write (to follow the verb in the question). If the essay question requires you to write an article review, for example, your response to the question will have to evaluate the merits of such a piece of writing. You will then need to produce an evaluative essay and you will signpost your introduction using verbs such as 'evaluate', 'judge', 'analyse', which will at the same time reflect the verb in the question (see the section on grammar and English use later in the chapter). These considerations will help you choose the best type of essay to answer the question you were given.

Remember that signposting the introduction will create certain expectations in your reader's mind, and it is your responsibility as a writer to make sure that these expectations are met in the rest of your essay. If, for example, you signpost your essay with:

This essay will examine the value of vaginal examination of pregnant women on hospital admission.

what expectations will your reader have? You have signposted an evaluation. You have told your reader that you will 'examine the value of something'. They will expect you to evaluate the worth of doing vaginal examinations when a pregnant woman is admitted to hospital. They will expect you to use words such as 'analyse' and 'examine'. They will not expect a description of how vaginal examinations are carried out on admission to hospital, for example. If you give such a description, your reader will be disappointed, because you failed to meet the expectations you created in their mind.

Similarly, if your introduction states that 'The essay will present a description of the latest medical technologies for the ICU' but your readers find a debate on ethical problems instead, they will feel dissatisfied. They were expecting to find a description, not a debate. Make sure that your essay has achieved what its introduction promised. Reader disappointment usually results from unmet expectations. And disappointment of this sort will result in a low mark for you.

The other important function of the introduction is to outline the content of the essay. The content of your essay is partly announced in the topic sentence, but mainly in the focus (see Chapter 1). However, it is always a good idea to wait until you have planned the body of your essay to outline the content in the introduction.

As you can see, the value of the introduction cannot be underestimated. The introduction will help keep you focused and organized. It will also serve as the map of the territory for the reader. It will show readers the path you have planned for them, and what content they can expect to find in the body.

The main body

What should the paragraphs in the body of an academic essay do? They should develop the focus and the rationale that you presented your reader with in the introduction. You will mainly accomplish this by presenting your supporting evidence in blocks of information (see also Chapter 1). Each of these blocks will deal with one issue as you signposted it in your introduction, and may require one or several paragraphs to do so.

Let us take the example about vaginal examinations. You may want to assess their value as (i) a method of measuring progress in labour, and (ii) a method of assessing abnormal presentations of the foetus. Then your reader may expect two fairly long body sections, each dealing with one of these. This is shown in Figure 2.3.

Body paragraphs

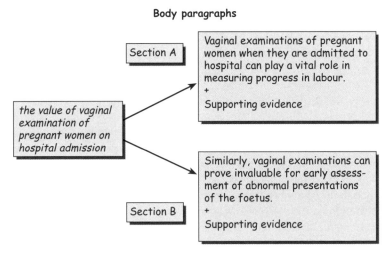

Figure 2.3 Body paragraphs in an essay

Let us look at another example of how to structure information in the body of an academic essay. Your introduction indicated: '*This essay will describe the latest medical technologies for the ICU. It will focus particularly on three of the most important – electronic charting, boom technology and dispensing systems.*' The body of your essay would then need one block for each of these technologies. For example, it could include one or more paragraphs on each of the following:

- Electronic charting on nurses' stations
- Boom technology
- Automated dispensing systems for pharmaceuticals.

In each of these blocks, you could support your claims by describing, but not arguing for or against, the main features of these technologies. You would need to describe what these technologies are and how they function, including enough information to cover them adequately. In this way, you will provide your reader with a fairly complete picture of the technological advances for critical care, while meeting the expectations you created in them.

The conclusion

What does the conclusion do? It summarizes or rounds off the main issues that you announced in the introduction and explored in the body of the essay. Apart from bringing together the issues presented in the body, the conclusion will normally draw the reader's attention back to the focus of the essay that was presented in the introduction (see also Chapter 1). This will create a sense of satisfaction in the reader. The expectations that your introduction creates in their mind are later met in the body of your essay, and finally rounded off in the conclusion.

Conclusions sometimes leave the reader with something to think about as well. However, you should be careful not to confuse this with new issues about the topic. Issues that are not announced in the introduction cannot be introduced in the conclusion. The conclusion is the part where you 'close doors' rather than open them.

Table 2.1 presents a checklist of things you may need to review after you have finished writing your essays. If your answer to any of the questions is 'no', you

Table 2.1 A checklist for the academic essay		
Questions	Yes/No	Action if 'no'
1. Have you chosen the best **type of essay** to answer the **essay question?**		
2. Have you presented the **introduction** clearly, indicating **topic** and **focus?**		
3. Have you signposted your **purpose** clearly (describe, explain, compare etc.)?		
4. Have you **structured** the body of your essay **effectively** (e.g. one main idea developed in each paragraph)?		
5. Have you **written enough** about the subject to cover the focus adequately?		
6. Have you supported your main ideas by **specific examples** or **evidence?**		
7. Have you included only **information** that is **relevant** to the topic and the focus?		
8. Have you included **enough details** in your supporting information?		
9. Have you concluded in a **logical** and **satisfactory** manner?		

should then decide what action you will take to improve that particular aspect of your essay. As you use the checklist more regularly, add new questions to it so that it becomes more relevant to your needs as a writer.

The academic essay may serve as the basis on which other genres can be planned and structured. You will probably have to make some adaptations to the basic structure. For example, in a longer essay you will have more paragraphs or more references to develop and support your information adequately. However, even longer essays will still show the basic structural elements: introduction, body and conclusion. The rest of the chapter explores longer genres such as the care critique, the review article and the argumentative essay.

ACTIVITY 2.1

Here are three essay questions and the introductions that have been written to answer them. As you read the introductions, try to evaluate how effective they are. Think of some reasons to back up your decisions. You may use these questions to guide you:

- Can you identify the **topic, focus** and **signpost** of the essay?
- Do they provide the reader with **enough information** to know what the text will be about?
- Can you say what you **expect to find** in the body of each of the essays?

Essay question 1

What does providing care for the critically ill patient involve? Discuss.

Introduction 1

Despite the great advances in medical treatments, many patients spend their final hours in intensive care units (ICU). More often than not, people are afraid of having a high-technology death with prolonged periods of suffering, and taxing obligations for their family. Caring for the critically ill patient in an intensive care unit then means that difficult ethical problems must be faced and resolved.

Essay question 2

Analyse the role of reassurance in nursing care.

Introduction 2

There are various roles that a nurse is supposed to carry out, and among the different personal qualities that these roles involve, reassurance seems to be the most important. Reassurance has been described as a powerful element to ease patients' fears, concerns and anxieties during their stay in hospitals. This essay will explore the concept of reassurance in connection with the patient's concerns and anxieties when hospitalized. It will first discuss some definitions of reassurance in an attempt to isolate its main attributes.

Essay question 3

Evaluate the value of models for treating dual-diagnosis clients.

Introduction 3

Dual-diagnosis specialists are becoming increasingly aware of the need to develop a treatment model that addresses the challenges posed by clients with severe mental health problems and a history of misuse of substances. There are a few intervention programmes to treat clients with a dual diagnosis. However, they are relatively new and have not been objectively evaluated for their effectiveness. In some countries, increasing attention is being paid to these issues and, as a result, several integrated-approach treatment programmes have been set up. These involve specialized multidisciplinary teams, working to address the unmet needs of clients. This essay will briefly describe the existing models and thoroughly examine their value. Against this background, the essay will evaluate the potentials of the new programmes in the light of the results obtained in their implementation.

Answers See suggested answers on p. *194.*

The care critique: an introduction

This section of the chapter presents an introduction to the care critique, one of the most frequent genres in nursing and midwifery. Because it is so important, we will take a closer look at it in Chapter 5.

Two terms normally associated with the care critique are 'criticize' and 'critique'. How do they compare?

- 'Criticize' is related to the bad qualities of something and to showing disapproval. It is normally based on what the speaker or writer dislikes or thinks is wrong or inappropriate.

- 'Critique', on the other hand, is associated with the writer's reaction to the value of something. 'To critique' means to present a balanced evaluation (what is good and bad) of what is being considered and 'a critique' is the essay you write when you do this.

Whereas criticism points out negative aspects, a critique analyses the value of something. The critique focuses on the object being analysed, rather than on the writer's subjective opinion or personal experience. In the care critique, the writer's focus of attention is the care, how effective, relevant and appropriate this care has proven to be, and the recommendations that s/he can make to improve the care provided.

The structure of the care critique will then show:

- An introduction, stating topic, focus and signpost.
- A body, identifying main issues in connection with the topic and clinical practice.
- A conclusion, summarizing main issues and showing their link with the focus.
- Recommendation/s (how care could be improved).

Activity 2.2 provides an example of how a care critique can be structured.

ACTIVITY 2.2

Read the essay question and the marking criteria. Then look at the outline for the care critique. Judging from the outline, how effective would you say the critique will be? Use the ratings provided below and be prepared to give reasons for your choice.

1 = Very effective; **2** = Effective; **3** = Not very effective; **4** = Not at all effective

Essay question: The role of the midwife in supporting a woman who chooses to smoke during pregnancy

Essay type: 3000-word care critique

Marking criteria:
1. Work neatly presented, easy to read and within the word limit
2. Clear identification of issues relating to care
3. Able to articulate theory and practice
4. Knowledge of basic concepts and issues
5. Accurate and appropriate referencing.

Outline:

Intro: Smoking during pregnancy, smoking cessation, statistics
         Midwife plays a fundamental role (informs, supports, helps to make informed
         decisions, provides alternatives)
         Care provided by an experienced midwife the writer has observed
         Essay will discuss support offered in terms of information and empowerment of
         the client

Body:
1. Present information about care provided
2. Identify issues (client's own choice, consequences for foetus, consequences for
   client etc.)
3. Information: How it was provided (explanation, materials, literature etc.)
                   What the midwife did with it
                   How the midwife checked information was understood and
                   processed by the client
4. Empowerment: How the information was used
                   How it helped the client make informed decisions
                   The results
5. Analysis: What was achieved by the midwife's intervention
                   What could also have been done
                   What was ineffective and why

Conclusion: Summarize main issues, draw attention to focus
   Make recommendations: How support could be improved

Answers *See suggested answers on p. **194**.*

The journal article review

Another typical genre in nursing and midwifery is the journal article review. This is
a critical account of a published article. It critiques the main aspects and the
contribution that the article makes to knowledge. In nursing studies, articles used
for review have normally been published in journals such as *Critical Care Nurse*,
Journal of the American Academy of Nurse Practitioners, *Journal of Nurse-Midwifery*,
Nurse Education Today and *Journal of Advanced Nursing*.

   The article review is normally between three and four pages long (between 800
and 1000 words) and it is a piece of academic writing. This means that you should
observe conventions of style, organization and presentation (see also Chapter 1),
as well as referencing conventions (see also Chapter 10).

   Although you will need some kind of description and, for this, you will use
descriptive language, the focus of your review should be on analysis and

evaluation. In an article review, you are expected to do more than describe the contents of the article. You must also analyse and evaluate the methodology and findings of the research.

Your review should show that you can:

- Think clearly and with originality.
- Think critically.
- Write concisely.
- Write academically.

There are four essential steps in preparing to write an article review, described in Table 2.2.

Table 2.2 Preparing to write an article review	
Steps	**Comments**
1. Draw up a list of questions to keep in mind while reading.	For instance 'Who wrote the article?' 'What are their credentials?', 'When was it published?', 'Where was it published?', 'Do its contents seem to be well researched?'
2. Read the article more than once.	It's important that you become familiar with the article you're about to review. Read it for general understanding first, and then read it again (and again if necessary) for its content, methodology and findings.
3. Read and take notes.	As you read the article for the second (or third) time, jot down things that you notice or that attract your attention (e.g. inconsistencies). You will need these notes for outlining your review. Remember, your review should *critique*, not only *describe*, the article.
4. Read and network.	As you read it for the last time, try to make connections between the ideas or issues in this article and those in other sources you have read. You can then compare the article with the sources that are related in topic or methodology when you write your review.

Let us now consider one possible way of organizing and structuring the review. This approach divides the review into five sections.

Section 1 gives the full bibliographical reference of the article: its author/s, title, journal name, volume, issue, year and page numbers.

Section 2 is the introduction. Here you should state the topic of the article and the thesis or main idea/purpose of your review. You should also include the audience for whom the article was written, and the assumptions the article appears to make about the readers' background knowledge.

Then, say something about the journal itself. Get a copy from your library and read the aims and scope of the journal so that you can say whether it is the appropriate journal for this particular article. Finally, mention what type of article this is. Articles can be classified into two types:

- The conceptual article: this supports its thesis mainly by means of logical and **persuasive reasoning.**
- The empirical article: this supports its thesis with substantial evidence, normally drawn from research studies.

Section 3 is the summary of the article. Remember to provide your reader with only the main points of the content and arguments within it. Your brief summary (no more than three paragraphs) should include:

- The problem being addressed.
- If available, the research questions that have prompted the author/s to conduct the experiment or write the argument.
- The solution being proposed and the evidence being provided.

Section 4 is the core of your review. This is the analysis. It is where you show how well you can evaluate the strengths and weaknesses of the article and how clearly you can define your position in relation to the author's. In this section, you should examine whether the article establishes a logical connection between the research questions introduced at the beginning of the article, the evidence presented in the body of the article to answer these questions, and the conclusions it reaches, based on that evidence.

Suppose that you were reading an article whose author had wanted to investigate the perceptions that a group of women in a given geographical area held about the care received postnatally. You would expect an article like this to be based on data collected from this specific population. You would expect it to describe research methods and data-collection instruments appropriate for 'capturing perceptions' (e.g. in-depth interviews). Then, depending on the data size, you would expect it to generalize results and draw conclusions that might apply to similar contexts. Judging whether it does these things satisfactorily would form the core of your review.

> **Glossary**
> Stance (as a writer or reviewer)

This section should also indicate your **stance** as a reviewer in a critical manner (also see Chapter 10). It should show:

- Whether you agree or disagree with the point/points made by the author.
- Your reasons for this.

ACTIVITY 2.3

Read the following introduction of an article review and decide if it is a good example. Here are some questions that may help you decide:

1   Does it include all the necessary bibliographical information?
2   Does it state the topic (of the article) and the purpose (of the review)?
3   Does it mention the audience of the article and the assumptions that the writer has made about them?
4   Does it refer to the journal as an appropriate forum for the article?
5   Does it mention what type of article this is?

Aston, J., E. Shi, H. Bullôt, R. Galway & J. Crisp. (2006). Quantitative evaluation of regular morning meetings aimed at improving work practices associated with effective interdisciplinary communication, *International Journal of Nursing Practice*.

This article reports on a research study that aims to evaluate interdisciplinary surgical morning meetings (SMM) at a ward of a major paediatric hospital. Such meetings were introduced to reduce communication and work-process problems among interdisciplinary professionals who provided care for children and their families. The article was written for nurses and doctors working in infants' and toddlers' hospital wards. The writers assume that their readers will not only have clinical experience in these wards but will also be aware of the problems of miscommunication and its implications for the children and their families. The journal is an appropriate choice for this empirical article as it publishes contributions that, according to its aims and scope, advance the 'understanding and development of nursing, both as a profession and as an academic discipline'. This review will provide a short description of the study and evaluate its contributions to the existing body of knowledge about interdisciplinary teams in acute-care environments.

Answers See suggested answers on p. 195.

- How any weaknesses you have spotted could have been avoided.
- Any assumptions that you believe affect the validity of the study.

This section will vary slightly depending on whether you are reviewing a conceptual or an empirical article. If you are working on a conceptual article, this section should include:

- An appreciation of its logic: do the different parts of the article contradict one other? Does the conclusion logically result from the introduction and the arguments in the body?

- A consideration of its coherence: does the line of reasoning follow a coherent development? Does each part naturally lead to the next?
- An analysis of the substance of the article: does the article shed new light on the issues it explores? Does it merely summarize previous knowledge or debates?

If you are reviewing an empirical article, you should then look at factors such as:

- Its clarity: does the article clearly develop its research question/s?
- Its literature review: where does the research connect with the existing literature?
- Its design: is this the most appropriate way to investigate the research question/s? Are the data-collection instruments well designed? How valid is the study?
- Its analysis of the data: are the statistics used appropriate for the type of data? Is the description of qualitative data sufficient to understand the analysis?
- Its discussion and conclusions: are the authors' claims clearly justified?
- Its ethical considerations and the biases of the authors: have the ethical issues been addressed? Have the authors done anything to minimize their own biases?

Section 5 is the conclusion. Here you sum up your position in relation to the article and indicate the contributions that the article makes to the field.

There are many different ways in which an article may contribute to advancements in its field. It may:

- Look at an old problem from a new perspective.
- Provide new results or shed new light on something old.
- Suggest new solutions.
- Present issues in such a way that the relationship between theory and practice is highlighted.

In the conclusion, you should not only state the contributions the article makes but also why you think those contributions are important or significant.

ACTIVITY 2.4

Using the questions in Activity 2.3 and the bulleted points used in various parts of this section, make your own checklist of the things that an effective review article should do. You can divide the checklist into introduction, body and conclusion, for example, which will also help you with the structuring of your own reviews.

The argumentative essay: an introduction

This section of the chapter introduces the argumentative essay. Like the care critique, this is a central genre in nursing and midwifery studies. It is what you will be doing in the later stages of your course, so we're going to look at it again in Chapter 6. Here, we will consider what argumentation is and analyse the logic and the structure of an argument.

As the cline in Figure 2.2 on page 23 illustrates, argumentation is different from description. Whereas description entails depicting what something is like or the facts about it (as in the 'room to let' ad), argumentation involves presenting a claim (sometimes called a *thesis*), supported by reasoning and evidence, in an attempt to convince readers that the claim or thesis presented is valid (as in the letter to the editor).

An academic argument is also different from a personal opinion in that the latter does not necessarily have to be supported by logical reasoning or evidence. If, for instance, you say: 'I don't like the way he treats his patients', you may not need to support your personal opinion with evidence. What is more, if challenged, you could simply say: 'Because I don't.' In academic argumentation, once you have made a claim, you need to use evidence to support it.

What is the logic of argumentation? When we plan an argument, we normally think about three things:

- What we assume to be true (e.g. nurses need to learn academic writing to advance their careers).
- Our conclusions based on our assumptions (e.g. nurses who can write academic pieces should be better off professionally).
- The evidence that supports both our assumptions and our conclusions (examples of nurses who have benefited from knowing how to write academically).

The logic of argumentation can be illustrated as in Figure 2.4.

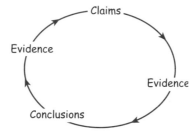

Figure 2.4 The logic of argumentation

It is important to mention here that each of these parts of the logic of an argument is dependent on the others. Our thesis will obviously affect our conclusions; if, after stating our thesis, we find evidence that challenges it, our conclusions will also be challenged. As we saw in connection with the article review, the logic of an argument should follow a coherent development and each part should naturally lead to the next.

As with other pieces of academic writing, when writing an argument you must plan your ideas first. This will help you focus your ideas and make sure that they are presented clearly and logically. Table 2.3 illustrates the typical organization and structuring of an argumentative essay.

Table 2.3 The structure of an argument	
Section	**What does it do?**
Introduction	States the aim of your essay, presents your claim or thesis, and mentions the reasons given to support your claim.
Statements	As well as including your supporting evidence, the statements discuss evidence that contradicts the argument.
Summary	Presents a brief review of discussion (supporting and contradicting evidence) and balances it, favouring your position.
Conclusion	Restates the views identified at the beginning of your essay, possibly discusses alternatives, examines implications of the conclusions, and/or makes recommendations based on the conclusions.

As you can see, the overall structure of the argumentative essay follows that of the general academic essay discussed earlier in the chapter. We will consider the argumentative essay in more detail in Chapter 6.

ACTIVITY 2.5

Read these two short texts. One is more descriptive than the other. Decide which is which, and think of reasons to justify your choice.

Text 1

Many arguments have been advanced in favour of the benefits of returning a patient with a stroke to the open-plan unit. These include the positive support reported by the patients and the quality of the follow-up care. However, the advantages of allowing patients with a stroke to stay in the same room have not been fully examined. Many patients with a stroke have reported that they would have paid for a private room for critical care. These patients could benefit from having the privacy for themselves and their families that a private room can offer. They could also profit from being closely monitored by the nurse stationed right outside their room.

Text 2

Equipping a room to the standards required for providing critical care involves making many decisions. After recovery, the patient will have to be allowed to stay in the same room. This will reduce patient transport and lower exposure to infections. Nurses' stations will have to be positioned outside the room for easy access and monitoring, while favouring patient privacy at the same time.

Answers See suggested answers on p. 195.

Grammar and English use

In this last section of the chapter you will find some suggestions about how to deal with grammar and language-use problems that many students experience when writing descriptive and critical pieces. If you need more detail on any of these topics, see the Glossary of Key Terms and the list of Further Readings and Resources at the end of the book.

The language of description

In Table 2.4 you will find words (verbs, adjectives and adverbs) that are frequently used in descriptions. You can use these words to talk about facts and describe what things or people are like. The table also shows the functions of these words (what you can use them for), their connection with academic writing (the types of writing in which you can use them) and some examples.

Table 2.4 Verbs, adjectives and adverbs frequently used in description			
Word class	Functions	Types of writing	Example
Relating verbs (e.g. be, have, there is, there are)	Definitions, describing features, providing details, making comparisons	Descriptive essays, record keeping, background information in a case or care critique, providing evidence, describing facts in an argument	The patient **was** administered 4000 U standard heparin intravenously before placement of an arterial cross-clamp at 9.32 am.

Action verbs (e.g. discover, report, show, state, compare, contrast)	Describing events, reporting, instructions, making comparisons, describing findings, describing graphs	Background information in a case or care critique, describing research findings, describing facts in an argument	The study **reported** an increase in the number of patients who self-refer to hospitals.
Describing words (e.g. essential, informed, static)	Making a description of a person or thing more precise	More precise description of a person or event	Midwives play an **essential** role in helping the **pregnant** smoker to make **informed** decisions.
Words that describe actions (e.g. well, slowly, hard)	Making a description of an action more precise	More precise description of how something was done	The information leaflets were given out to patients **appropriately**.

The language of argumentation

In Table 2.5 you will find verbs and adverbs that are frequently used in writing in critical genres such as the article review, the care critique and argumentative essays. The table shows the functions of these words and some examples.

Table 2.5 Verbs and adverbs frequently used in argumentation

Word class	Functions	Example
Acknowledging verbs (e.g. admit, recognize)	To admit limitations or incompleteness	We have to **admit** two main limitations in this study.
Comparing verbs (e.g. correspond to, compare with)	To draw a comparison between ideas or arguments	His position **compares** favourably with that of his predecessors.
Emphasizing verbs (e.g. insist, reiterate, remark, stress)	To provide emphasis to a point/idea in an argument, or the argument itself	She **insists** that these are fundamental considerations relating to clinical care.
Establishing verbs (e.g. demonstrate, prove, solve, fail)	To establish that someone or something has or hasn't been successful at demonstrating something	This has **demonstrated** that not all patients favour moving to an open-plan unit after they have recovered.
Positioning verbs (e.g. claim, hold the view, recommend, suggest)	To show the writer's position, discuss it and/or challenge it	This seems to **suggest** that the writer considers that most of these events could have been prevented.
Emphasizing adverbs (e.g. convincingly, conclusively, definitely, forcefully, successfully)	To emphasize how something was done	They have **forcefully** made the case that units should be fully equipped to provide the best possible care.

Revising the objectives of this chapter

Tick those objectives that you feel you have achieved and review those you have not yet managed to accomplish. Then, complete the **Achievement Chart** at the back of the book.

In this chapter, you have learnt to:

☐ recognize the difference between description and argumentation

☐ identify the main academic genres in nursing and midwifery

☐ understand the purpose and the structure of these academic genres

☐ identify the main language items used in descriptive and critical writing.

Processes in Academic Writing

At the end of this chapter, you should be able to:

- recognize the nature and stages of the reflective process
- identify different critical thinking processes
- understand the principles of the critical evaluation of evidence
- identify key language items used in reflective and critical writing.

Reflection and the reflective process

Chapters 1 and 2 laid down the foundations of academic writing. Chapter 1 explored three basic issues in academic writing: planning, organizing and paragraphing; and Chapter 2 built on those principles to deal with more specific genres such as the care critique, the journal article and the argumentative essay. This chapter considers reflection and critical thinking, two specific processes that you will need to write in other genres such as the reflective essay covered in Chapter 4. The chapter begins by exploring the nature and stages of the reflective process and then moves on to analyse the principles of critical thinking.

In this section of the chapter, you will analyse reflection as a concept and as a process.

Let us start by looking at some phrases connected with reflection as a concept. Complete the spidergram in Figure 3.1 with three words or phrases that you usually associate with 'reflection'. One has been given as an example.

Figure 3.1 Spidergram

You probably included ideas such as 'learning from past experience', 'evaluating what happened', 'applying practical wisdom', 'examining what was done', 'getting better prepared for the future' and 'empowering'. All of these ideas have to do with reflection.

Simply defined, reflection means learning from what you do so that you can be better prepared for the future. Through reflection you can learn to change aspects of yourself, your professional practice, or both. Reflection can be seen as a bridge that connects past and present experiences to decide what future actions you need to take (Durgahee 1996).

Donald Schon (1987) distinguished between 'reflection-on-action' and 'reflection-in-action'. Reflection-on-action is about looking back at an experience or event. Reflection-in-action is associated with thinking about something while you're still doing it.

In this chapter you will be concerned with **reflection-on-action** – that is, with examining a past event so that you can learn how to do better in the future.

Reflection-on-action

This learning experience has three aspects to it, matched by three action stages, as illustrated in Table 3.1.

Table 3.1 Aspects of the learning experience	
Aspect	Action
Reflexivity: looking at how 'self' has developed throughout time	You revisit or describe a past event or experience and think about the people involved in it.
Understanding: gaining insights as to how and why things happened	You examine what happened, why it happened and how it could be done differently.
Empowerment: being able to change things in the future	You then decide on a course of action that will help you do things better next time.

Figure 3.2 shows the reflection-on-action process. Notice that the reflective process is cyclical rather than linear. Today you revisit yesterday's events, but tomorrow you will need to revise today's experiences. This is the essence of reflection as a process for professional development and as the basis for becoming a reflective professional.

Figure 3.2 **The reflection-on-action cycle**

Reflection-on-action examines past events or experiences from a critical perspective. Remember that it is a learning experience that aims to improve the weaknesses in the professional practice of the person who reflects.

This means that reflection is a *critical* and *evaluative* process. It is not a *descriptive* process. This critical and evaluative process is clearly manifested in the reflective essay, which we will discuss in more depth in Chapter 4.

Let us now examine the different stages of reflection-on-action as outlined above.

Researchers have put forward many conceptual models of reflection-on-action. The three best-known models are those developed by Van Manen (1977), Gibbs (1988) and Durgahee (1996). Van Manen's is a general model that details reflection as a process for professional advancement. It includes three different levels of reflection: the evaluation of a given performance, the analysis of its consequences and the critical examination of its associated issues.

Both Gibbs' and Durgahee's models work at a more practicable level. Gibbs' model is probably the most widely cited in nursing and midwifery. It comprises the following stages:

- Description: what happened, what your feelings were at the time.
- Evaluation: what was good and bad about the situation.
- Analysis: what sense you can make of it.
- Conclusion: what else could have been done.
- Action: what you would do next time around.

Durgahee divides reflection into three levels:

- Macro level: the actual recall of the experience.
- Meso level: the identification of its associated issues.
- Micro level: the understanding of the experience based on feelings and personal views.

As with most conceptualizations, these models have their limitations; however, they represent three strong theoretical frameworks for developing the critical skills needed for reflection.

For each of the three stages in the reflection-on-action process that you saw in Figure 3.2, there are some **critical skills** that you will need to develop. These critical skills are highlighted in italics in the following description of the reflective process:

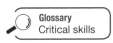

Glossary
Critical skills

- The **first stage** involves not only explaining the experience and issues identified in it but also *exploring preconceptions* and *assumptions* about it.
- The **second stage** analyses what happened and the reasons why it happened, but also deals with *questioning/challenging the preconceptions* revisited in the first stage.
- The **third stage** is the actual reflection, by which you not only examine what has been learnt and what needs yet to be learnt, but *identify learning needs* and *plan concrete actions* to resolve future conflicts.

Let us analyse the critical skills involved in each step in more depth. After explaining the main issues that resulted from the experience you revisited in the first stage, you need to explore the preconceptions and assumptions made at the time of the experience. It is important to notice here that exploring preconceptions and assumptions does not mean finding a justification for them, but rather producing an objective analysis of what lies behind them.

The second stage involves challenging these preconceived ideas. Are they still valid? Do they need to be modified? If they do, how can they be modified? What would be the most appropriate way of modifying the preconceived ideas identified? This stage is more analytical in nature than the first one.

The third stage is the most critical. In this last stage you should adopt an objective perspective on the experience and on your feelings about it, making a connection between what you have learnt from this and the actions that you plan to take in the future.

Table 3.2 summarizes the issues involved in each of the three stages and the skills that the student in Activity 3.1 would need to reflect on the experience. The numbers in brackets refer to the stages; the reflective skills required are in italics and given in square brackets. How does this table compare with the answers you provided in Activity 3.1?

ACTIVITY 3.1

Read the following short case and think of how the student involved in it could reflect on the experience. Then complete the chart with your ideas on the issues she should identify at each stage and the reflective skills needed for each of the stages.

On her first clinical placement, a student nurse was asked by her placement supervisor to care for a client in a wheelchair. She hadn't done this before and she wasn't sure she could manage. Nevertheless, she decided not to tell her supervisor that she had no experience with anyone in a wheelchair. She was asked to take the client to radiology for an x-ray. Before pushing the chair, the student wanted to make sure that the client had her feet on the foot rest. She pushed the foot rest into position and, without realizing, she hurt the client's leg.

Stage	Issues to identify	Critical skills needed
1. Explaining and exploring	Explaining the experience:	Exploring preconceptions/ assumptions:
2. Analysing and challenging	Analysing what happened and why; how it could have been different:	Challenging preconceptions/ assumptions:
3. Examining, identifying and planning	Examining what has been learnt:	Identifying learning needs/planning actions:

As the examples in Table 3.2 show, key questions can help you go through the different stages to identify the reflective skills that you need to use in each stage. Some of these questions have been presented here, but you may wish to add more or develop your own set.

Table 3.2 The reflective stages		
Stages	Issues	Skills
Stage 1: Explaining and exploring	What happened? (1) 1. It was the first time the student had to provide care for a person in a wheelchair. 2. The student did not say how she was feeling about the request.	What assumptions did they make? (1) [exploring assumptions] • Supervisor: The student knew what to do and how to do it. • The student: She could eventually handle the task.

LIBRARY, UNIVERSITY OF CHESTER

JET LIBRARY

Stages	Issues	Skills
	3. The wheelchair footrest hurt the client's leg. **Context (1)** 4. The student's first clinical placement. 5. The hospital ward, the radiology department. **Who was involved? (1)** 6. The placement supervisor 7. The student nurse 8. The client	
Stage 2: Analysing and challenging	**Why did it happen? (2)** 9. The student didn't tell the supervisor she had never provided care for a person in a wheelchair. 10. The supervisor failed to check. **Could it have been done differently? (2)** 11. Yes, the supervisor could have taught the student how to handle the situation.	**Did the assumptions prove right? (2)** [challenging assumptions] • For the supervisor? • For the student nurse? **Do the assumptions need to be changed? (2)** • Do the supervisor's assumptions need to be changed? If so, how can they be changed? • Do the student's assumptions need to be changed? If so, how?
Stage 3: Examining, identifying and planning	**What should the student have learnt from this experience? (3)** 12. Effective communication is extremely important in caring for patients. 13. Decisions should be informed and based on knowledge and experience.	**What does the student still need to learn? (3)** [identifying learning need] • To express her feelings, especially when she is doing something for the first time. • To get support when she is doing things she feels she is not fully trained for. • To gauge the possible consequences of her actions. • To learn to make more informed decisions. **Future action (3)** [planning concrete actions] • To learn ways of expressing feelings. • To get trained in handling and moving patients.

The principles of critical thinking

Being able to reflect on your practice is an important part of the broader process of becoming a critical thinker. In this part of the chapter we will look at the principles of critical thinking and see how you can develop your own critical thinking abilities. Being a good critical thinker means that you can assess the arguments presented by other people to see if they are logical, well thought out, and properly supported with relevant evidence. It is an ability that you can use when you read as well as when you listen to someone presenting a point of view or proposing a course of action.

Stella Cottrell (2017, p. 2) defines critical thinking as 'a complex process of deliberation which includes a wide range of skills and attitudes'. This implies that you can identify these skills and evaluate how good you are at each of them so that you can improve any weak areas.

When you are assessing someone else's arguments, good critical thinking includes being able to:

- Identify other people's positions, arguments and conclusions.
- Evaluate the evidence for alternative points of view.
- Weigh up opposing arguments and evidence fairly.
- Draw conclusions about whether arguments are valid and justifiable, based on good evidence and sensible assumptions.

When you are writing an essay or presenting your point of view, critical thinking allows you to lay out an argument in a structured, clear, well-reasoned way that convinces others.

These skills and attitudes can be seen to fall into three different phases that are essential to the critical thinking process: **identifying, evaluating** and **presenting**.

These phases may seem linear, but in actual practice they may occur more than once in a cyclical manner. For instance, you may need to revisit the position that other people have put forward as you realize that some of the assumptions on which their argument was based are false.

What does each of these phases involve?

Phase 1: Identifying positions, arguments and conclusions

To recognize people's positions, you will need to identify:

- How they position themselves in their argument.
- What positions of others they endorse or do not endorse.
- What possible biases their arguments present.

The way in which people use language can provide you with valuable help to recognize their positions. Some questions you can use to discover a writer's or speaker's position, for example, include:

- Are they positioning themselves as part of the issues analysed? As an insider? Or an objective outsider? What grammatical person (e.g. he, she, they) do they use? What grammatical structures (e.g. impersonal 'it') do they employ?
- What does the writer or speaker agree with? What do they disagree with? What verbs do they use to mark endorsement or lack of it (e.g. these authors have advanced influential…, these writers have ignored…)?
- Does the writer/speaker recognize his/her own biases? Does s/he use language that indicates this (e.g. I intend to follow…)?

Identifying people's arguments at this stage is also connected with how they structure the information in these arguments. You need to identify the claim that serves as a starting point for their argument, how their claim is supported and what conclusion or conclusions they draw as a result (see also Chapter 6).

Consider, for example, the following claim in an article on encouraging pregnant women to stop smoking:

Smoking cessation during pregnancy is unsuccessful because support to the pregnant woman is only occasional and lacks structure.

If you identify this as the writer's main argument, you should expect a critique of current systems of support, based on evidence. You should also find some conclusions and recommendations about how smoking cessation during pregnancy can be made more effective. Coupled with this structural recognition, you should also identify some strategies that can make the writer's argument more persuasive. Some of these strategies involve:

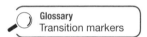

Glossary
Transition markers

- Presenting the opposing argument first.
- Using **transition markers** that indicate an opposing view (e.g. 'however', 'nevertheless'), which can also help highlight the writer's own argument.
- Contrasting the weaknesses of the first argument (usually the opposing argument) with the strengths of the writer's argument.

Phase 2: Evaluating evidence and arguments

This is a central stage in the critical thinking process. Here, you need to consider whether the writer or speaker has presented a balanced picture by offering evidence both to support and to counter his/her views. Other important aspects to consider are the value of the evidence used, whether the logic of the argument is flawed, and whether the conclusion is logical. Some questions you can use to evaluate evidence and arguments include:

- Does the writer present a balanced picture of the issue/s by including opposing views and arguments? How balanced is the presentation?
- How strong is the evidence presented to support the claims being made? Is it closely related to the argument? Or is it only indirectly linked? Is it practice-based? Is it research-based?

● Is there a logical relationship between the different parts (claim, evidence and conclusion) of the argument?

● Does the conclusion develop logically from the issues explored and the evidence presented?

Phase 3: The presentation of the argument

This phase is crucial for evaluating other people's arguments. Like identifying, presenting combines structural as well as logical elements. The logical elements are connected with how well reasoned and well balanced the argument is. The structural elements have to do with the clarity and the structure. Questions to examine the presentation of an argument may include:

● Does the presentation contribute to persuading the reader that the argument is valid?

● Are the arguments presented in a well-thought-out and clearly planned manner?

● Does the presentation follow a logical order?

● Does the writer use language effectively to support his/her logical order (e.g. using connectives such as 'first', 'finally', 'on the other hand')?

ACTIVITY 3.2

● Applying the three phases of critical thinking (identifying, evaluating and presenting), analyse the following short text. Can you recognize any of the critical strategies discussed so far? Use some of the questions suggested for each phase to help you.

● Many studies have produced inconclusive evidence in relation to the efficacy of the support that smokers receive during pregnancy (e.g. Kelley *et al*. 2001; Melvin *et al*. 2000; Melvin & Gaffney 2004). Several of these studies suggest that brief interventions do not significantly contribute to smoking cessation during pregnancy (Fiore *et al*. 2000; Lumley *et al*. 2004). Lawrence *et al*. (2005, p. 115), for example, have forcefully concluded that 'in-pregnancy programmes may have immediate benefits to the foetus, but do not influence the smoking outcomes of mothers in the medium term'. This seems to indicate that smoking cessation in pregnancy is unsuccessful because support to the pregnant woman is only occasional and lacks structure. Programmes of sustained support would need to be implemented so as to help smokers not only during pregnancy but also after giving birth. These programmes should then be structured in such a way as to offer both in-pregnancy and post-partum support. Combined strategies have been suggested as a successful element of these programmes. Some of the in-pregnancy strategies may include providing information leaflets on the risks of maternal smoking to the foetus and the infant, helping to set a quit date, and teaching cognitive and behavioural strategies for stopping. After-pregnancy strategies should include control of the levels of nicotine, provision of rewards and peer support groups.

Answers See suggested answers on p. 195.

Critical analysis of evidence

In the previous section you examined how to identify a writer's or speaker's claims and purpose, and how to evaluate the consistency and worth of his/her arguments. Another important skill in critical thinking is being able to evaluate the sources of evidence that someone has used to support their argument. Although this critical analysis is important for all kinds of sources of evidence, it becomes of paramount importance when you have to examine internet-based sources (see Chapter 1).

In this section, you will examine two different, though interrelated, ways of evaluating sources. You will first look at the *quality* of the sources and then at their *relevance*.

Determining the quality of the sources used to support an argument is fundamental, as their quality will determine the quality of the argument itself. Sources in an argument are like the foundations in a house. If the foundations are not properly laid, the rest of the structure may collapse (also see systematic reviews in Chapter 7).

Typical questions you may ask when analysing the *quality* of the sources used to support an argument include:

- Who wrote the material? What professional affiliation do they have? Have they written on the subject before? Are they cited by others?
- When was the evidence published?
- In the case of evidence found in books, is the book a new edition? Has the new edition been (substantially) revised?
- Who published the material?
- What kind of publication is it? Is it an internationally known journal? Is it a local newspaper?
- Who was the material written for? Who was its intended audience? Was it written for the general public?
- Was the content presented in a well-reasoned manner? Are there flaws in the argument?
- How much does the content cover (breadth and depth of coverage)?
- What contribution does the content make to the issue/s being discussed?

The *relevance* of source material is related to the importance of the information for developing the writer's claims. The questions you need to ask to examine the relevance of the sources include:

- Are the claims and supporting evidence closely related? Are the claims too general?
- Does some of the evidence challenge the claims?
- Is the evidence strong enough for the writer to have a case?
- Does the conclusion develop logically from the claims and the supporting evidence?

Look at the following sources of evidence. Can you evaluate them in terms of their quality? You will need to do a library or internet search to find more information about them before you can decide on their quality. Use the suggested questions in the chapter if you need guidance.

1   Maslin-Prothero, S. (Ed.) (1997). *Baillière's study skills for nurses*. London: Baillière Tindall in association with the Royal College of Nursing.
2   Lawrence, T., P. Aveyard, K.K. Cheng, C. Griffin, C. Johnson & E. Croghan. (2005). Does stage-based smoking cessation advice in pregnancy result in long-term quitters? 18-month postpartum follow-up of a randomized controlled trial. *Addiction*, 100(1), 107–16.
3   Evaluating sources of information. *Online writing lab*, Purdue University. Available at http://owl.english.purdue.edu/owl/resource/553/1/. Last accessed on 23 March 2018.
4   Spiegel, R. (2004). *Psychopharmacology: An introduction*. 4th edn. Chichester: John Wiley & Sons, Ltd.

Answers See suggested answers on p. 196.

Reflection and critical thinking are cognitive processes that require the use of specific language and grammar when you need to talk or write about them. The process of reflection, for instance, requires that you keep the right sequence of tenses when you refer to the past event on which you are reflecting, your present reflection and the future actions you intend to take. Similarly, critical thinking tends to be associated with certain verbs such as 'analyse' and 'synthesize' and certain structures that you can use to show your stance as a writer. These issues are explored in the next section.

Grammar and English use

In this section you will find suggestions about how to deal with some grammar and language-use problems that many students have when employing reflection and critical skills. If you need more detail on any of these topics, see the Glossary of Key Terms and the list of Further Readings and Resources at the end of the book.

Verbs connected to 'reflection'

Table 3.3 shows you some verbs that recur when discussing reflection. It also shows associated words that you can use, for instance to avoid repetition or create cohesion in your texts (see Chapter 1). Some examples of how you can use them are also given.

Table 3.3   Verbs frequently used in reflective texts

Verb	Common accompanying words	Example
Assess	*Noun*: assessment *Adverbs*: accurately, correctly, fully, properly *Similar words*: appraise, evaluate, estimate	Reflecting on the experience provided her with an opportunity to **assess** the situation in the ward accurately.
Assume	*Noun*: assumption *Adverbs*: naturally, reasonably, safely *Similar words*: presume, suppose	She first **assumed** that nurses were familiar with the side effects of all drugs.
Attend to	*Noun*: attention *Adverbs*: continually, carefully *Similar words*: deal with, take care of	In the first place, it was necessary to **attend to** every one of her needs continually.
Challenge	*Noun*: challenge *Adverbs*: effectively, forcefully, seriously, (un)successfully *Similar words*: contest, question	Her initial assumptions were seriously **challenged** by the facts she later collected.
Evaluate	*Noun*: evaluation *Adverbs*: carefully, continually, critically, fully, properly, systematically, thoroughly *Similar words*: assess, estimate	His assumptions were systematically **evaluated** against the sources associated with smoking cessation during pregnancy.
Explore	*Noun*: exploration *Adverbs*: carefully, briefly, extensively, fully, systematically, thoroughly *Similar word*: inspect	In the second stage, they had to **explore** all the possible alternatives before they could make a final decision.
Identify	*Noun*: identification *Adverbs*: accurately, clearly, (in)correctly, positively *Similar words*: distinguish, single (out)	It is essential to **identify** the assumptions lying behind one's own actions.
Involve	*Noun*: involvement *Adverbs*: actively, directly, inevitably, typically *Similar words*: entail, include	The problem **involves** all people connected with his care: his nurse, his social worker and his family.
Perform	*Noun*: performance *Adverbs*: adequately, effectively, efficiently *Similar words*: accomplish, achieve	You can learn a great deal from examining in retrospect how your peers **performed**.
Plan	*Noun*: plan *Adverbs*: carefully, intelligibly, meticulously, systematically *Similar words*: chart, project, map (out)	Based on your own past learning experiences, you can carefully **plan** further actions to be better prepared for the future.
Reflect on	*Noun*: reflection *Adverbs*: fully, thoroughly *Similar word*: think	This essay will **reflect on** the most central issues associated with primary care.

Tense sequence for reflection

When writing a reflective essay, keeping the right sequence of tenses (present, past, future) may prove problematic. Below are some key things that you should remember about tense sequence.

Present descriptions: Present time in real situations (not hypothetical or imaginary ones) can be described by:

- Simple present – The morning shift for nurses **starts** at 6.00 a.m.
- Present progressive – The patient **is being** diagnosed.

Present tenses are normally used to describe the event or situation on which we want to reflect. How these tenses combine depends on the logical sequence of events. For example, the present perfect (e.g. have gone, has decided) has a connection with the past (an action that started some time in the past) and usually means that the action is not finished. It may be necessary as background information to a present event:

> He **has been taken** to the operating room where he **is being operated** on for tendon rupture.

Present descriptions tend to connect with the future by means of the future simple tense (will):

> After the nurses finish with the admission routine, the patient **will** be sent to the A&E unit.

Past recounts: Past events can also be described by a number of past tenses:

- Simple past – The treatment **was** a success.
- Past progressive – They **were organizing** the patient's records when they were called to a staff meeting.
- Past perfect – They **had finished** completing the admission form when the patient collapsed.

In some cases two past actions can be described by using the simple past without creating confusion in the reader. For example:

> The nurse **managed** to finish the admission form before the patient **collapsed**.

This is usually the case when you use words such as 'before' and 'after' to join the two actions. But notice the difference in meaning between these two versions of the same example:

> (1) The nurse **had finished** the admission form when the patient **collapsed**.
> (2) The nurse **finished** the admission form when the patient **collapsed**.

The past perfect (*had finished*) in (1) is used to indicate that this is the first of the two actions. The simple past (*finished*) in (2) is used to indicate that both activities happened at almost the same time.

To indicate future in the past we use 'would' instead of will:

The doctor thought the patient's heart **would** not restart.

Future actions: Actions in the future can be expressed by:

- The simple future – They **will** finish their midwifery programme in six months.
- The present progressive to indicate an arrangement – I **am seeing** my placement supervisor next week.
- 'Going to' to indicate a future plan – The student **is going to** get some training in handling and moving patients.

Verbs connected to 'critical thinking'

Table 3.4 shows you some verbs used in connection with critical thinking, words that are commonly associated with these verbs (collocations) and some examples.

Showing your stance

A writer's stance can be defined as his/her position in relation to the subject matter of his/her writing and how he/she relates to the audience. (Also see 'reporting verbs' in Chapter 10.) For example, in a sentence like 'helping women make informed decisions is a fundamental aspect of the role of the midwife', you can see that the writer views the subject matter (helping women make informed decisions) as an essential part of the midwife's role. In a sentence like 'Most readers will certainly appreciate the importance of effective communication in providing nursing care for patients', you can see that by addressing the audience directly (*most readers will*) the writer is establishing a relationship with them. Also, if you carefully look at the writer's choice of words (*most, certainly, appreciate, importance, effective*), you can see how the writer relates to the subject matter. Similarly, you can show how you interpret other people's stance as writers by the verb you use to report their words. If, for example, you write 'Brown (2004) says that...' you are just reporting but not interpreting Brown's words, as you are when you write 'Brown (2004) denies/criticizes/suggests that...'.

Thus, 'showing your stance' as a writer means showing how certain you are about what you're claiming, how you feel about it or how strongly you support or challenge someone else's opinion. Here are some examples of how you can show your stance:

1 The results of the study **are** inconclusive.
2 The results of the study **seem** inconclusive.
3 The results of the study **may seem** inconclusive.
4 The results of the study **might look** inconclusive.

Sentences 1–4 show different degrees of certainty, from most certain to least certain. That is, they show how positive you are about the claim you're making. By using words or phrases such as 'seem', 'may', 'probably', 'appear to be', 'might', you can indicate a more tentative stance than when you use the verb 'to be' for instance, as in 1 above.

Table 3.4 Verbs frequently used in critical texts		
Verb	Connected words	Example
Analyse	answers, arguments, evidence, ideas, methods, preferences, relationships, theories etc.	This essay will **analyse** the relationship between these two aspects.
Be	accurate, active, analytical, consistent, evaluative, logical, open-minded, precise, rational, systematic etc.	Their argument **is a systematic** attempt to end world poverty and ill-health.
Differentiate	attitudes, facts, fallacies, ideas, opinions, truth etc.	It is important to be able to **differentiate** facts from opinions.
Draw	attention, conclusions, distinctions, inferences, lessons, plans etc.	Its ultimate aim is to try to **draw** lessons from these changes.
Evaluate	accuracy, arguments, assumptions, authenticity, beliefs, evidence, viewpoints, worth etc.	He has always been good at **evaluating** the authenticity of other people's claims.
Identify	arguments, ideas, differences, positions, similarities etc.	The next section of this critique will **identify** the differences and similarities between the two methods.
Interpret	meanings, experiences, information, results, significance, sources etc.	They failed to **interpret** the results of the study in the light of the research questions posed at the beginning of their article.
Weigh up	advantages, (opposing) arguments, disadvantages, risks etc.	Risks should always be **weighed up** against the benefits that clients may get.

5   The **deadly** virus has reached continental Europe.

Adjectives (e.g. deadly) and adverbs (e.g. forcefully) give the reader an indication of where you stand in relation to the facts described. In sentence 5 above, the writer is showing his/her position in respect to the spread of the virus.

   Your choice of verbs also shows your position as a writer with regard to other people's ideas or arguments. Notice the difference in 'strength' of support to what others have expressed given by 'suggest' in 6 and 'confirm' in 7:

6 Brown (2003) **suggests** that the contradictory results in these two studies have been produced by the different research methods used.
7 Ellis (1994) **has confirmed** that women who suffer from post-partum depression find support groups extremely useful.

Another way of showing your stance is by referring to previous work that has influenced yours, establishing similarities and differences between them, as shown in 8:

8 This essay follows Gibbs' pioneering examination of reflection as the basis for professional development. Unlike Gibbs', the present framework, however, aims to ...

Revising the objectives of this chapter

Tick those objectives that you feel you have achieved and review those you have not yet managed to accomplish. Then, complete the **Achievement Chart** at the back of the book.

In this chapter, you have learnt to:

☐ recognize the nature and stages of the reflective process

☐ identify different critical thinking processes

☐ understand the principles of the critical evaluation of evidence

☐ identify the key language items used in reflective and critical writing.

Writing in Genres in Nursing and Midwifery

This second part consists of four 'how to' chapters that will help you apply the principles of academic writing that you examined in Part One. In this part, you will study how to write a reflective essay, a care critique, an argument and other common nursing and midwifery genres: the action plan, the care plan, the portfolio, the report, the systematic review and the research proposal.

CHAPTER 4: HOW TO WRITE REFLECTIVE TEXTS

Reflective writing is often the first type of writing that nursing and midwifery students are required to do. This chapter will show you how to apply the theoretical principles outlined in Chapter 3 to write reflective essays and accounts of performance.

CHAPTER 5: HOW TO WRITE A CARE CRITIQUE

Chapter 5 focuses on the process and the product of critiquing. It starts by examining what is involved in writing a care critique and how it is organized and structured. It then shows how the final product should reflect the critique of the care in its conclusion and recommendations.

CHAPTER 6: HOW TO WRITE AN ARGUMENT

This chapter opens with exercises to help you differentiate between opinion and argument. It then presents practical ways of identifying the strength of an argument, followed by considerations about structuring arguments effectively. Finally, the chapter identifies the main language items that are commonly used in argumentative writing.

CHAPTER 7: HOW TO WRITE IN OTHER GENRES

Chapter 7 introduces other common genres that you may be required to master. The chapter first examines action plans, care plans, and research proposals and portfolios. It then focuses on personal diaries and academic and professional reports. The chapter moves on to analyse systematic reviews, case studies for assessment purposes, and the research proposal that you will have to present for your dissertation. Finally, it explores how to plan and get organized to write an undergraduate dissertation.

How to Write Reflective Texts

At the end of this chapter, you should be able to:

- plan a reflective essay appropriately
- identify an effective way of introducing reflective essays
- recognize the structure of body paragraphs to support introductions
- recognize ways of producing an effective conclusion
- write effective reflective accounts of performance
- identify the style of the reflective essay.

Planning the reflective essay

In Chapter 3 you analysed the nature and the structure of the reflective process. In this chapter, you will examine how this process can be used to plan a reflective essay. The reflective essay is an analytical piece of writing. This means that when you write a reflective essay, you need most of the reflective and critical skills you examined in Chapter 3. It also means that description will be used as background information, although it will not be the focus of a reflective essay.

Let us start by drawing a comparison between description and reflection based on two experiences on clinical placement. Read the main differences between these two processes as illustrated in Table 4.1.

When planning a reflective essay, you will find it useful to devise a table like Table 4.1, where you can list the main differences between description and reflection in relation to the experience you want to analyse. As this table shows, description is concerned with the factual – the reality around the experience. Reflection, on the other hand, has to do with evaluating the event so that it becomes a learning experience.

Your reflective essay will have to combine the description of the facts that made up the event or experience with your 'reflective evaluation' of it. Remember, however, that description will be a small part of the reflective essay. It will only be used to set the scene or provide the background information on which your

Table 4.1 Description vs reflection		
Past experience	Description	Reflection
A student nurse on a recent clinical placement	The physical environment where he was (the ward, the beds, the clients), who he talked to (supervisors, clients, nurses, other students), what he did (what he was told or asked to do)	How he felt at the time, what he learnt from the experience, what he discovered he didn't know, what perceptions he had before the placement (were they confirmed/challenged?), what he plans to do about his needs, what skills he has developed/needs to acquire
A student helping a midwife with a breastfeeding educational campaign	The physical environment where she was (the room, the clients), who she interviewed, what the midwife did with the women, what was said, the procedures followed	How she felt about the experience and the procedures, what she learnt, her assumptions at the time, what she needs for her development as a future midwife

evaluation will rest. You will have to describe the event, but you will also need to demonstrate what you have learnt from it and how.

Here are some further steps that you will want to consider when planning the structure of your reflective essays:

- Examine the essay question.
- Read the marking criteria if available.
- Identify the event or experience on which you will reflect.
- Make sure that you maintain the anonymity and confidentiality of the patients, clients, staff and institutions involved.
- Jot down notes that briefly describe the experience (you can draw up a table here or draw a mind map or a concept map).
- Make a note of the main issues you have been able to identify in relation to the experience.
- Think of ways in which you can relate these main issues to the literature (sources).
- Jot down some further notes that reflect your understanding of the issues identified, and the insights you gained from the experience.
- Think of ways in which you can relate insights you have gained to the literature (sources).
- Make notes as to how you will make the connection between theory and practice clear.
- Note down how you plan to discuss your future personal and professional development needs.

These structural points will show your reader that after the experience you:

- have developed into a more reflective person (reflexivity);
- have gained new insights (understanding); and
- are now able to change things for the future (empowerment).

ACTIVITY 4.1

Read the following account of a past experience that a student midwife went through. Use the chart beneath to differentiate between description and reflection in the account.

A mother's perception of milk insufficiency seems to be one of the most common reasons for discontinuing breastfeeding. As a student, I assisted a midwife in providing care for Isobel, a primigravida, two days after normal delivery of her baby. We visited Isobel in her home, a terraced house in the Borough of Haringey, London. Isobel had become very anxious about breastfeeding as she reported that her baby did not seem to be getting enough milk and demanded to be breastfed all the time. Isobel felt that she needed to start complementing her breast milk. Having made sure that the baby was latching on properly, I told the client that it was normal for some babies to require to be fed all the time. As a way of building the mother's confidence and to avoid discontinuing breastfeeding, the midwife explained to her the supply-and-demand nature of breast milk. Isobel needed to have as much information as possible to make informed decisions. This would also help to lower her anxiety level. This made the writer realize the importance for new mothers of getting consistent supervision and breastfeeding advice.

Experience	Description	Reflection

Answers See suggested answers on p. 196.

Examining introductions

In Chapter 1, you examined the basic elements in essay introductions. This section of the chapter will analyse other possible elements in the organization and structure of introductions in reflective essays. Remember that introductions are a fundamental part of any essay, as they represent the map of the territory that the reader will explore.

When readers of your reflective essay finish reading your introduction, they should also be able to answer the four basic questions for any type of essay:

- What is the essay about?
- What exactly does the essay focus on?
- Why is it important to analyse this?
- How will it be developed?

You may sometimes need to include other pieces of information in the introduction, especially when you are writing a longer essay. Apart from the information provided by the answers to these four questions, your introduction may also need to include:

- A **transition** between the topic and the focus. When the topic is too broad and the focus too narrow, you will need to add one or two transition sentences to make the text flow more smoothly.
- **Definitions** of terms. When you use terms that are controversial or on which consensus has not yet been reached, you will need to define exactly how you will use them.
- **Reference** to models. In the case of the reflective essay, you may need to state the model of reflection (e.g. Gibbs 1988) that you will follow.

Glossary
Transitions/Transition markers

Let us consider two examples of introductions that include these other pieces of information. The first example includes a definition (**D**), a transition (**T**) and a reference to a model (**M**). The second example includes a longer transition (**T**). The first develops the question:

What have you learnt from your recent clinical placement?

and the second answers:

How has your experience in helping the professional activity of a midwife enabled you to develop new insights?

EXAMPLE 1: INTRODUCTION

Reflection has been identified as an extremely useful skill for nurses (Durgahee 1996; Johns 1996; Mountford & Rogers 1996). Schon (1991), for example, defines reflection as learning from events during a practical professional experience (**D**). Clinical placements also offer a unique opportunity for learning through reflection (**T**). Following Gibbs' (1988) cycle of reflection (**M**), this essay will discuss two areas that the writer has been able to identify as needing development for his future professional activity. The first of these is knowledge of the multidimensional nature of pain. The second relates to pain-assessment tools, especially in relation to post-operative pain.

EXAMPLE 2: INTRODUCTION

Reflection is considered an appropriate vehicle for the analysis of professional practice. This analysis helps professionals understand the nature of their work and adopt a critical approach to their professional activity (Gould & Masters 2004). Student midwives can also learn from reflecting on the professional practice of others when, for example, they shadow a midwife on their daily practice on the ward (**T**). This essay reflects on the insights gained in helping the professional activity of a midwife. It first explores the nature and process of reflection. It then examines how reflection has provided the basis for developing new insights into professional midwifery practice. The essay finally recommends future actions to enhance the development of the professional skills of the student midwife.

Reflection and the body of the essay

The reflection process will find its home in the body of your reflective essay. This means that the body of the reflective essay will contain the different stages of the reflective process that we examined in Chapter 3. It will present:

- A description of what happened and what your feelings were at the time.
- An evaluation of the experience or event (what was good and bad about it).
- Your analysis of the experience (what sense you can make of it).

It is always a good idea to make explicit use of a reflective model. For instance, Gibbs' reflective cycle (see Chapter 3) is a popular model that encourages a description of a past situation, analysis of feelings, evaluation of the experience, and an examination of what you would do if the situation arose again. You may use this model for your reflective essay, but you will have to use more analysis in each of its stages if you are writing at level 3 or Honours level.

Another possible model is the framework for reflexive practice (Rolfe *et al.* 2001), based on Driscoll's model (1994). This framework is based on three questions – 'What?', 'So what?' and 'And now what?' – that are supposed to stimulate reflection at different levels. The first question should start you reflecting on the situation for you to be able to describe it. The second question encourages you to construct a personal theory about the situation and to learn from it. The third and, according to the developers of the framework, the most important stage should help you consider how you can improve the situation and the consequences of your own actions. Yet another model is Johns' (2004) model of structured reflection. This model can be used for general reflection on experience as well as for analysing more complex processes such as a critical incident, making it ideal for analysis at level 3 or Honours level.

Let us look at one concrete example of planning and structuring the body of the reflective essay following Gibbs' model. Notice how analysis permeates each paragraph of the body section. Here is the question for the reflective essay, followed by the marking criteria:

How have your clinical knowledge and skills developed to help you meet the requirements for registering as a nurse?

The marking criteria given for this essay are:

- Work clearly presented, easy to read, free from spelling and grammar mistakes.
- Shows ability to reflect on own knowledge and skills, identifying main issues and problems associated with professional practice.
- Demonstrates ability to make a clear link between theory and practice.
- Can make connections between requirements for registration and knowledge and skills developed.
- Shows ability to integrate evidence-based support from the literature.
- Demonstrates capacity for identifying future needs.
- Accurately referenced following academic conventions (see Chapter 10).

Here is one possible way of planning and structuring the information in the body of the reflective essay in reference to the essay question and the marking criteria above. You have been given the outline for the introduction so that you can see the relationship between the body and the introduction:

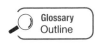
Glossary
Outline

- **Introduction** – introduce topic (what?): how can the requirements for registration be met; the focus (what exactly?): main requirements for registration are principles behind client-centred care, understanding of culture-sensitive practices, literacy and numeracy skills; signpost (how?): reflecting on experiences on course and on clinical placements.

- **Body section 1**: Topic: principles related to client-centred care. Requirement for registration, how principles developed (literature), how theory informed clinical practice and vice versa (literature), what has been learnt from reflection (connection with experience), identification of future needs.
- **Body section 2**: Topic: culture-sensitive practices. Requirement for registration, how understanding developed (literature), how theory informed clinical practice and vice versa (literature), what has been learnt from reflection (connection with experience), identification of future needs.
- **Body section 3**: Topic: literacy. Requirement for registration, literacy development (literature), how theory informed clinical practice and vice versa (literature), what has been learnt from reflection (connection with experience), identification of future needs.
- **Body section 4**: Topic: numeracy. Requirement for registration, numeracy development (literature), how theory informed clinical practice and vice versa (literature), what has been learnt from reflection (connection with experience), identification of future needs.

Notice how planning the essay following the organizing principle presented in the introduction (general to specific) has contributed to its structure. The paragraphs in the body develop the main issues identified in the focus of the introduction and the issues have been developed in the way that was signposted in the introduction.

Reflection and the conclusion of the essay

Conclusions serve the purpose of bringing the essay to a satisfactory end. This means that your conclusion should show the relationship between the different parts of the essay (see Chapter 1). The conclusion of a reflective essay will then:

- Provide a summary of the issues explored in the body of the essay.
- Remind the reader of the main purpose of the essay.
- Suggest an appropriate course of action in relation to the needs identified in the body of the essay.

The introduction and the body of the reflective essay presented in the previous section can be concluded by:

- Summarizing the main issues identified.
- Drawing the reader's attention to the focus of the essay (principles behind client-centred care, understanding of culture-sensitive practices, literacy and numeracy skills).
- Identifying a course of action that links back to the needs identified in the body paragraphs.

Reflective accounts of performance

This section of the chapter deals with reflective accounts that you will be asked to write of your performance in an individual or group presentation.

ACTIVITY 4.2

Read the following conclusion that has been written following the outline above. Has the conclusion been developed in an effective way? Be prepared to give reasons to support your answer.

Client-centred care is one of the basic principles that a nurse should learn to provide. It conceives of the client as a holistic individual. This principle should form the basis of both the theory and the practice of nursing care. To provide client-centred care, nurses should be able to recognize culture-sensitive practices and the way these are related to social cultures in general (Papalexandris 2004). Societal characteristics are important sources of information for nurses to be able to make informed decisions in their daily practice. Informed decisions will obviously be the result of reflection on practice and respect for ethnicity, culture and differences.

Answers See suggested answers on p. 196.

As we have already discussed in relation to reflective essays, it is important to decide which reflective model you will use for writing your account of performance. Also as suggested before, either Gibbs' (1988) or Driscoll's (1994) model can help you structure your account. Table 4.2 shows a possible way to structure an account of a presentation based on Gibbs' model of reflection.

You can also use the questions provided in Driscoll's model to guide you as to the content of each of the sections in your reflective account. Table 4.3 shows how you can combine the categories in Gibbs' model and some of the questions in Driscoll's.

Table 4.2   A possible structure for an account of a presentation

Stage	Contents	Recommendation
Description	Here you briefly describe what happened during the presentation. This will provide readers with the necessary background information in order to understand the sections that follow.	Keep it short, as it is meant just to set the scene for the rest of your account.

Stage	Contents	Recommendation
Feelings	Describe here what you were thinking and feeling as the presentation was being delivered.	Include only those aspects of the presentation that you will reflect on later. This will keep your account tight and relevant.
Evaluation	Analyse what was good and bad about the presentation.	Produce an objective and balanced account, including both strengths and weaknesses of the presentation. Remember also to analyse what was good and bad rather than just describe it.
Conclusion	Explain here the outcome of the presentation and mention what else could have been done in the situation.	It is important for you to emphasize what you think could have been done differently, as this will pave the way for the action you are planning on taking, which is the next section in your account.
Action plan	What would you do for your next presentation?	Remember to refer here to both what you would keep because it was successful and what you would improve next time around.

Table 4.3 Categories and questions for reflection on performance	
Categories	Questions
Description	What is the purpose of returning to this situation?
	What happened?
	What did I see or do?
Feelings	How did I feel at the time of the event?
	Were those feelings different from those of other people involved in the event?
	Have my feelings about the event changed?

Categories	Questions
Evaluation	What were the effects of what I/we did or didn't do?
	What positive aspects now emerge from the event?
	What have I noticed about my behaviour in practice?
Conclusion	What implications can be drawn from the event?
	What could have I/we done differently?
	What difference would it make if I chose to do nothing?
Action plan	How can my/our performance be improved?
	Which aspects should be tackled first?
	What is the main learning that I/we can take from this?

Grammar and English use

In this last section of the chapter we will analyse the style of reflective essays and accounts of performance. Figure 4.1 shows some common problems and how to solve them. If you need more detail on any of these topics, see the Glossary of Key Terms and the list of Further Readings and Resources at the end of the book.

Table 4.4 Style problems in reflective essays and accounts of performance		
Problem	Solution	Examples
The use of personal pronouns It may seem appropriate to use personal pronouns, especially 'I', to refer to personal experiences on placement. However, the use of personal pronouns may be distracting for the reader, drawing their attention to the writer rather than to the experience being analysed.	Change the focus of attention Make the experience and what you have learnt from it the focus of your writing.	Original: I will reflect on my experience with a double-diagnosis patient during my clinical placement. Improved: This essay will reflect on the writer's clinical experience with a double-diagnosis patient.

Problem	Solution	Examples
The use of contracted forms Contracted forms (e.g. isn't, haven't, I'll etc.) are representative of informal speech. Remember that a reflective essay is a piece of formal writing.	**Spell out all contractions** Use full words (is not, have not, I will etc.) rather than contracted forms.	**Original:** The patient wasn't prepared for the event as he hadn't been told about it. **Improved:** The patient was not prepared for the event as he had not been told about it.
The use of informal language Similarly, informal language is commonly used in other non-academic genres (e.g. personal letters).	**Use formal language** Formal language is careful and accurate language, characterized by formal vocabulary and impersonal structures.	**Original:** I kind of know what it is but I can't really say much about post-operative pain, you know. **Improved:** Post-operative pain is a difficult concept to define and requires a precise approach.
Unsupported claims Unsupported claims are usually accepted in spoken genres and when you want to present or discuss your personal opinions.	**Use references from the literature** In academic writing, every substantial claim that you make should be supported by some form of evidence (e.g. references from books, journal articles etc.).	**Original:** Many have talked about the importance of communication in nursing for a long time. **Improved:** The importance of communication in nursing has been at the centre of professional debates for many years (Atkinson 1985; Smith 1990; Orr 2004).

Revising the objectives of this chapter

Tick those objectives that you feel you have achieved and review those you have not yet managed to accomplish. Then, complete the **Achievement Chart** at the back of the book.

In this chapter, you have learnt to:

☐ plan a reflective essay appropriately

☐ identify an effective way of introducing reflective essays

☐ recognize the structure of body paragraphs to support introductions

☐ recognize ways of producing an effective conclusion

☐ write effective reflective accounts of performance

☐ identify the style of the reflective essay.

How to Write a Care Critique

At the end of this chapter, you should be able to:

- define the care critique
- plan and organize the care critique effectively
- structure the main sections of the care critique
- provide effective conclusions and make sensible recommendations.

Pre-reading task

Re-read the section on the care critique in Chapter 2 before reading this chapter.

Defining the care critique

In Chapter 2, we considered the basic elements of a care critique. In this chapter, we will examine how to structure and organize the care critique in more depth.

Before considering the organization and structure of a critique, let us explore words or phrases that you associate with a 'critique'.

A critique requires presenting a balanced evaluation of what is being considered. For this, you will need all the reflective skills examined in Chapter 3. Thus, words such as *analytical thinking* and *evaluative* are closely associated with a critique.

ACTIVITY 5.1

Put a tick (✔) next to the words or phrases that you consider are related to a 'critique' and a cross (✘) next to those that you think are not related. Then draw arrows to join the central balloon with those you have ticked.

Answers See suggested answers on p. 197.

ACTIVITY 5.2

Considering what you have learnt in Chapter 2 and your choices in Activity 5.1, how would you define a 'care critique'?

_____

_____

_____

_____

_____

_____

How does your definition compare with the one given below?

*A care critique is a **systematic, critical** and **impersonal** analysis of the care provided that discusses its **validity** and evaluates its **worth**.*

The words in bold are central to this definition of a care critique and merit further comment. Let us start with the first three: **systematic**, **critical** and **impersonal**.

'Systematic' refers to doing something in a coherent, thorough and principled way over a given period. Suppose that you want to examine systematically the care that patients who have had a minor accident receive after being discharged from hospital. You will first have to decide what is understood by 'care' and 'minor accident'. You will also need to examine this care over a given period, and focus on a patient who meets the criteria specified. Put together, these three elements represent examining the care in a systematic way.

'Critical', as we examined in Chapter 3, is related to being able to:

- Identify the position or view of the people involved in providing and receiving the care (i.e. what the professionals who provide the care think about it, and what the patients who receive the care think about it).
- Evaluate the reasons for providing the care and whether they were valid or not.
- Present a given point of view (probably based on the reasons or views of the professionals and the patients).

'Impersonal' refers to both your position on what you are analysing (not personally involved or attached) and the language that you use to represent the object of your analysis (e.g. employing impersonal language and structures).

The other two words, **'validity'** and **'worth'**, are closely connected with the verb 'to evaluate'. As you saw in Chapter 1, this means to determine the significance of something, usually by careful appraisal and study. In this sense, for your readers to realize the significance of the care, you will have to provide them with the positive and negative aspects of the care given. Based on the negative aspects you examined, you will have to then provide some recommendations (see later in this chapter).

To recap, a care critique is a systematic analysis of the care given to a patient. It is not a subjective recounting of the facts, but an objective evaluation of the care with recommendations for better practice.

Planning and organizing the critique

Now that we have defined a care critique so we know what it is, let us deal with what it does. A care critique has five essential aims. It should:

- Identify aspects of good practice in the care provided.
- Identify and outline a well-defined problem in the care being considered.
- Analyse issues in the care and data that can be used as evidence.
- Provide a solution or solutions to the problem.
- Demonstrate what action needs to be taken if necessary.

As you can see, there are five main verbs that indicate the purpose of a care critique. Let us analyse these verbs more closely:

- **Identify**: recognize something so that you can say who/what it is.
- **Outline**: give a brief description of the **main facts or points**.
- **Analyse**: examine the nature or structure of something in order to provide a **better understanding** or an **explanation** of it.
- **Provide**: make something available in a way that **can be used or put into practice**.
- **Demonstrate**: show something clearly, providing support, proof or evidence.

You need to remember something very important here: the basis for your analysis is *identifying*. If you don't identify the problem, none of the rest is possible. It is also important that you *outline* the problem for which the care was provided, rather than describe it in detail as you would do in a case study. Remember that the focus of the critique is the care provided and not the problem itself. The problem serves as background information to the care and is usually outlined in the first part of the body of the critique.

Once you have identified and briefly described the problem or issue, it is time for you to focus on the central aims of the care critique: analyse the issues, provide solutions and recommend a course of action.

Table 5.1 is a generic structure that you could use to plan and organize your care critiques. Whenever you have to write a care critique, you can use the right-hand column to jot down your own ideas about the contents.

Table 5.1 A generic structure for a care critique	
I. Introduction	
Topic (Go back to the care critique question)	
Focus (Issues you want to raise in connection with the care; connect issues with the learning outcomes of the module)	
Aims (What will your critique specifically do? How will it do it?)	
II. Body	
Contextualize the care (Brief description of the patient, the context, the need for care and what was done)	
Identify good practice (Highlight aspects of good practice in the care)	
Identify and outline the problem	
Issue 1 (Identify the issue and the sources you will use as support or evidence)	
Issue 2 (Identify the issue and the sources you will use as support or evidence)	
Issue 3 (Identify the issue and the sources you will use as support or evidence)	
III. Conclusion	
Summarize the main points	
Revisit your focus	
Discuss the validity/worth of care	
Make recommendations (to resolve problems/issues addressed in the body)	

Note that the 'body' section contains three issues. This is because in a typical 2000-word critique, you can only cover three or four related issues with a degree of depth. In longer pieces you could have more. However, you will always have to strike a balance between width and depth. Too many issues will require more words for you to deal with them in appropriate depth.

Structuring the care critique

Once you have finished planning the contents of the care critique, you will need to structure its information.

ACTIVITY 5.3

Read the following introduction of a care critique and identify the functions of the different sentences. Then fill in each of the bubbles with one of the labels provided.

① Identifies a well-defined problem

② States the focus clearly (issues)

③ Anchors topic in context

④ Signposts action by the care critique

In the UK there is wide recognition of the increasing number of patients with mental health problems who also misuse psychoactive substances. These substances range from alcohol, tranquillizers, barbiturates, heroin and stimulants such as amphetamines, cocaine and its derivatives, to cannabis and hallucinogens. Substances like these have an effect on the central nervous system in terms of altering moods, thought processes and behaviour. The combination of substance misuse and mental health problems is associated with a host of serious social, behavioural, psychological and physical problems, resulting in increased demands on mainstream services. As a result of their mental and health conditions, these dual-diagnosis patients face losing contact with friends, family and their homes. This critique will examine the care given to ten dual-diagnosis patients during the writer's clinical placement. More specifically, the critique will focus on the main factors that lead patients to lose contact with friends and family and the actions leading to the minimization of such loss.

Answers See suggested answers on p. 197.

The main sentences in this introduction serve very specific functions (or moves) that indicate to the reader the way in which the information is going to be dealt with in the rest of the text. As you probably realized in Activity 5.3, there are generic functions that readers will expect to find in your introduction:

> **Glossary**
> Generic
> functions

- Locating the topic in the general context of the discussion.
- Identifying examples of good practice.
- Identifying a well-defined problem and its main issues.
- Stating the focus of the critique.
- Signposting what the care critique will do.

As you saw in the generic structure presented above, the body of your care critique will then develop the issues you have identified in the introduction. The basic functions of the body of a critique are to:

- Present an objective summary of the care.
- Identify instances of good practice.
- Identify a problem or problems with the care.
- Establish the main issues associated with the problem.
- Critically discuss these issues using research-based evidence (e.g. references).
- Demonstrate what it is appropriate to do about the identified problem and its associated issues.

Concluding and making recommendations

The last section of the care critique is the **conclusion** (see also Chapter 1) and **recommendations**. This section of the critique should show three moves:

- Restate the identification of the problem.
- Summarize the main issues.
- Recommend a course of action that will improve the care being critiqued.

To write conclusions that wrap up the contents of the care critique in a satisfactory manner, you should take the following into account:

- When you restate the problem, focus on why this problem is **relevant** in the context of the care.
- When you summarize the main issues, state their **significance** in relation to the problem critiqued.
- When you make recommendations, revisit the **weaknesses** of the care.

ACTIVITY 5.4

Read the following example of a conclusion of a critique that examines the care provided to a woman in the third stage of labour. Considering what you have learnt about conclusions so far, how effective do you think this conclusion is? Give reasons for your answer.

This care critique has analysed the midwifery care given to Mrs M, during the third stage of labour. The period following delivery of a baby should be a time of relief and joy for all those involved. However, this period holds great potential dangers for the mother. Post-partum haemorrhage (PPH) has been identified as one of the main complications of the third stage, which accounts for the highest maternal mortality and morbidity. As demonstrated in this care, there is compelling evidence that lends support to the benefits of active management of the third stage as it decreases complications and morbidity, especially in high-risk cases. There is strong advocacy for prophylactic syntocinon administration during delivery of the baby and other medications commonly used in the active management of the third stage of labour as well as for CCT with counter-traction when the uterus is well contracted. There is also strong support for planning in advance and active management.

Answers See suggested answers on p. 198.

The recommendations that you make have to be connected with the body and the conclusion of the care critique. Recommendations should establish a **logical relationship** with the issues addressed in the body of the critique and should **sensibly result** from the conclusion that you have presented. Figure 5.1 represents this connection.

Figure 5.1 **The relationship between conclusion and recommendations**

The text in Activity 5.5 illustrates the type of recommendations that you could make to go with the conclusion presented in Activity 5.4 above.

ACTIVITY 5.5

How appropriate would you say that the recommendations made here are?

Midwives must be able to identify women at high risk, and make plans for emergency management so as to be prepared to deal with complications in a timely and systematic manner. It is recommended that clear and effective guidelines be provided to all midwives as well as training incorporated to support midwives in making the best possible decisions.

Answers See suggested answers on p. 198.

Table 5.2 presents a checklist of things that you should consider after you have finished writing your care critique. Remember to plan some action to improve those aspects of the critique to which you have given a negative answer. Add new questions to the checklist as you use it more regularly.

Table 5.2 A checklist for the care critique		
Questions	Yes/No	Action if 'no'
1. Have you presented the **introduction** clearly, indicating topic, focus and comment?		
2. Have you **structured** the body of your critique **effectively** (e.g. developing one issue in each section)?		
3. Have you presented an **objective summary** of the care provided?		
4. Have you clearly **identified the problems** with the care and their associated issues?		
5. Have you presented the **issues** in the body of your critique in a **balanced** and **comprehensive** manner?		
6. Have you supported these issues by **specific examples** from clinical placement and **evidence** from the literature?		
7. Have you demonstrated what would be **appropriate to do** about the identified problem?		
8. Have you shown why this problem is **relevant** in the context of the care?		
9. Have you stated the **significance of the issues** explored in relation to the problem critiqued?		
10. Have you **recommended a course of action** that will improve the weaknesses of the care critiqued?		
11.		
12.		

Grammar and English use

In this last section of the chapter, you will find information about the most common connectives used in academic writing. Connectives are words (e.g. 'and', 'but', 'so') or phrases (e.g. 'on the one hand') that are used to connect ideas, sentences or longer texts. If you need more detail on any of these topics, see the Glossary of Key Terms and the list of Further Readings and Resources at the end of the book.

Connectives can be used to provide cohesion (sticking together) to texts (see Chapter 1) at different levels. You can use connectives (see Table 5.3) to provide cohesion between ideas in (1) the same sentence, (2) different sentences and (3) longer pieces of writing, as these texts illustrate:

(1) The patient was in cardiac arrest **and** was assisted by an automated defibrillator.
(2) This kind of support has proved very effective in helping pregnant smokers cope with cravings. **On the other hand**, it has not had lasting effects after childbirth.
(3) Many arguments have been advanced in favour of the benefits of returning a patient with a stroke to the open-plan unit (Brown 1999; Thompson 2004; Willis 2002). These include the positive support reported by the patients and the quality of the follow-up care. **However**, the advantages of allowing patients with a stroke to stay in the same room have not been fully examined (Allen 2001).

Table 5.3 The use of connectives		
To	**You can use**	**For example**
add an idea	and, also, as well as, furthermore, in addition, next, another, other…	**Another example** of the complex relationship between…
add an opposing idea	but, however, on the other hand, in contrast, although, nevertheless, on the contrary, conversely…	**On the other hand**, this attitude has attracted a great deal of opposition from…
add a similar idea	Similarly, likewise, also, as, once again…	**Also**, we have to consider how many other possibilities lie…
give an example/ examples	For example, for instance, as follows…	We could say, **for instance**, that these reasons have not been well…
express exceptions or reservation	Even though, still, yet, nevertheless…	They have been widely researched. **Yet** the results provided by most studies…
give an alternative	In other words, or rather, alternatively…	**In other words**, we can go on like this for ever and ever.
identify a cause	For, because, since, as…	**Because** they didn't have all the necessary people in their team, they couldn't finish the project in time.
give an effect	Therefore, thus, hence, consequently, as a result, so…	They couldn't finish the project in time, **so** part of their fees…
list ideas in time order or order of importance	First, second, third etc., then, next, finally…	**First**, the essay will present an overview of…
mark a transition	Now, as far as X is concerned, with regard to, as for…	**As far as time is concerned**, I would like to make the following observations.

To	You can use	For example
make a generalization	In general, on the whole, in most cases, usually, frequently, mainly...	**On the whole**, these cases show that most patients would prefer...
highlight	In particular, especially, particularly...	**In particular**, this section of the dissertation will focus on...
give a summary or conclusion	In summary, to conclude, in short	**In short**, these are the three main issues that...

Revising the objectives of this chapter

Tick those objectives that you feel you have achieved and review those you have not yet managed to accomplish. Then, complete the **Achievement Chart** at the back of the book.

In this chapter, you have learnt to

☐ define the care critique

☐ plan and organize the care critique effectively

☐ structure the main sections of the care critique

☐ provide effective conclusions and make sensible recommendations.

How to Write an Argument

At the end of this chapter, you should be able to:

- recognize the difference between opinion and argumentation
- identify the strength of an argument
- structure arguments effectively
- identify the main language items used in argumentative writing.

Pre-reading task

Re-read the section on the argumentative essay in Chapter 2 before reading this chapter.

Evaluating claims

Read the two statements in Figure 6.1. Which states an opinion? Which one presents an argument?

Many professionals would now agree that the results of research in midwifery care are inconclusive and even contradictory.

A

Previous studies have shown that results of midwifery care research are inconclusive and sometimes contradictory (Kirkham, 2002; Powell Kennedy & Shannon, 2004; Raisler, 2000). However, recent research has demonstrated that ...

B

Figure 6.1 **Which is the argument?**

Whereas statement A sounds very formal and authoritative, and may even look like a claim, it is nonetheless an opinion. There is no evidence that supports the statement, so we can say that statement A simply states what the speaker or writer assumes to be true. Statement B, on the other hand, is a statement of a fact supported by evidence. As you read in Chapter 2, opinion claims do not necessarily have to be supported by evidence. You can say 'nursing is a difficult profession' and do not need to provide evidence of that. However, evidence is important in argumentation, as it is the basis on which your argument will rest. If

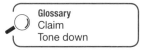

Glossary
Claim
Tone down

you express an opinion, there is then no argument, unless your opinion is challenged and you need to support it using evidence. Only then will you have an argument.

There are some questions that you can use to check whether the claim you are reading or making is a statement of opinion or an argument. Consider:

- Can you identify a clearly defined position taken on the topic?
- Have alternative positions been provided?
- Is there a call to action (e.g. a recommendation)?

If two answers to these questions are negative, then you have an opinion in front of you. Use the questions to check statement A above, for instance. There is no *clearly* identified position; there is only a vaguely stated idea. Similarly, no alternative positions have been provided and no action has been called.

Here is another list of questions. You can use these to challenge an argument. These questions should help you measure the strength of a claim, and thus also enable you to discern opinions from arguments.

- Does the claim reflect the writer's belief? If so, is the belief supported by other evidence-based arguments?
- Does the claim present evidence that both supports and contradicts it?
- How are the claim and the evidence related? Closely or only indirectly?

Apart from these questions, you may also think of the logic of argumentation in order to evaluate claims. What is the logic of an argument? Any **claims** will start with what the writers think or believe to be true. But this is an opinion. To make this claim a fact, they will need to provide **evidence**. Based on this, writers can then present their **conclusion** or **conclusions** about the fact or facts they have expressed. Now, you must make sure that their conclusions result from both the evidence and the claims they have made. The relationship between these three elements in the logic of arguments was illustrated in Figure 2.3 in Chapter 2.

Remember the following:

- **Analyse the thesis:** if the starting claim (thesis) is faulty, the whole argument is. Sometimes the thesis needs to be toned down as it does not always apply. For instance, the thesis may claim that a certain situation applies to (all) women in labour, but the evidence exemplifies only primigravida women. In this case the thesis needs to be toned down.
- **Analyse the relationship** between the presupposition, the supporting evidence and the conclusion. Watch out for particular instances and general claims, and inconsistencies in the relationship between the three.
- **Examine the conclusion:** the conclusion must logically develop from the thesis and the supporting evidence. Sometimes the claims are acceptable but the conclusion drawn from them is not.

ACTIVITY 6.1

Analyse the following statements and decide whether they are claims stating opinions (OP) or facts (FA). Be prepared to support your choices.

1   It has, for example, been suggested that whereas health promotion programmes at the national level have successfully met their targets, at more local levels similar programmes have failed to accommodate the needs of a growing population.

2   Previous studies have strongly supported the initiative of helping pregnant women stop smoking. However, some of these studies have produced inconclusive evidence in relation to the efficacy of support programmes for pregnant smokers (e.g. Kelley *et al.* 2001; Melvin *et al.* 2000; Melvin & Gaffney 2004).

3   We would argue that there is an ever-growing need for needs analysis exercises to determine the real needs of local populations in relation to midwifery health promotion.

4   Management of diabetes is improved if appropriately trained practice nurses are involved.

Answers See suggested answers on p. 198.

The strength of an argument

A strong argument will not only support its claims by providing evidence-based examples or support, it will incorporate and challenge opposing arguments, showing their weaknesses and how these could be solved.

One way in which you can work with opposing arguments is by analysing them vis-à-vis your own thesis. It is a good idea to start by making a list of the strengths and the weaknesses of the opposing arguments, so that they can be compared with the strengths and weaknesses of your own arguments.

Table 6.1 illustrates how the comparison between two opposing arguments can be charted. This will not only help you see how the two arguments compare, but also how you can use them to structure your texts, as we shall discuss in the next section.

Table 6.1 Argument comparison table			
Topic: The role of technology in the intensive care unit (ICU)			
Argument A: technological approach to ICU (e.g. Ray 1987; Benner *et al.* 1992)		Argument B: techno-ethico-human approach to ICU (Walters 1995; Alasad 2002)	
Strengths	Weaknesses	Strengths	Weaknesses
S1. The importance of technical aspects	W1. The effects of technology on ICU nurses have been ignored	S1. Focuses on the effects that technology can have on critical care nurses	W1. De-emphasizes the importance of technical skills in nurses
S2. The importance that ICU nurses give to care in this context	W2. ICU nurses have been seen as technical agents	S2. Follows a techno-ethico-human caring model	

Table 6.1 shows how the weaknesses of one argument can be related to the strengths of the other. For example, the first weakness of argument A (the effects of technology on ICU nurses has been ignored) can be contrasted with the first strength of argument B (focuses on the effects that technology can have on critical care nurses). If you had to write an argument using these claims, you could then produce something like:

The role of technology in the intensive care unit (ICU) has been the focus of a debate which has intensified in the last decade (Ray 1987; Benner *et al.* 1992; Walters 1995; Alasad 1992, 2002). Some of these studies have followed a technological approach to issues relating to the ICU. They have mainly emphasized the importance of the technical aspects of the ICU and of the significance given to the care by critical care nurses (e.g. Ray 1987; Benner *et al.* 1992). However, they have ignored the effects of technology on ICU nurses and have shown a tendency to see critical care nurses as technical agents. This study advocates a change of emphasis from technology to ethics, following what has been recognized as a techno-ethico-human model of care (Walters 1995; Alasad 2002).

The structure of argumentation

As we have examined in previous chapters, planning is a central activity in writing. This also applies to writing arguments. Planning will help focus your ideas and make sure that they are presented clearly and logically. The following guide will help you think through the planning process and structure your work clearly when writing argumentative texts (see also Table 2.3 in Chapter 2).

ACTIVITY 6.2

Based on the information in the following text, complete the argument comparison table beneath.

An essential first step in pressure ulcers prevention is the identification of those patients who are truly at risk. Since the early 1960s a variety of risk assessment scales (RAS) have been developed with over 20 such instruments currently described in the worldwide literature (Torra I Bou 1998). These scales assign numerical values to various patient traits (such as their level of mobility) with a total score generated from the sum of these values. Considerable attention has been given to comparison of different scales based on statistical constructs such as their sensitivity and specificity (Cullum *et al.* 1995; Anthony *et al.* 2000). However, such activity is subject to a major limitation: when risk has been identified preventive interventions are initiated, and so the 'true' sensitivity of any RAS cannot be measured. (Papanikolaou *et al.* 2002, pp. 187–188)

Topic: Risk assessment scales for preventing pressure ulcers	
Argument A (FOR)	**Argument B (AGAINST)**
Strengths	Weaknesses

Answers See suggested answers on p. 198.

- **Introduction**: What is the topic of your argumentative essay? What is its aim? What claim(s) do you want to make in it?
- **Main points**: What reasons will you give to justify your claim(s)? What reasons will you give to support your conclusions?
- **Supporting statements**: Apart from including your supporting points, what other points that contradict or place doubt on the argument will you discuss? How will you balance your statements?

- **Summary**: How will you review your discussion? What points will you highlight? How will you highlight them?
- **Conclusion**: How will you call the reader's attention to the main issues identified in your introduction? Will you include a brief discussion of alternatives for the future? How will you examine implications of the conclusions? Will you make recommendations based on the conclusions you presented?

ACTIVITY 6.3

Analyse the following text and decide how you could turn it into an argumentative text.

Many professionals would now agree that the results of research in midwifery care are inconclusive and sometimes even contradictory. It has, for example, been suggested that whereas health promotion programmes at the national level have successfully met their targets, at more local levels similar programmes have failed to accommodate the needs of a growing population.

Answers See suggested answers on p. 199.

Structurally an argumentative text should include these four elements:

1 A statement of the topic.
2 Argument or arguments that contradict the thesis.
3 A transitional marker denoting a contradiction.
4 A statement of the thesis.

The structure and organization of these elements in a text are illustrated in the short text by Jenkins and Elliott (2004, p. 623) in Figure 6.2.

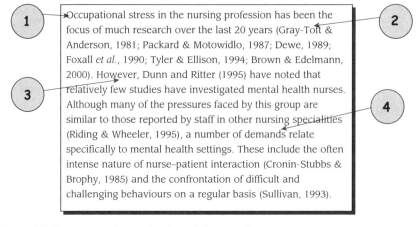

Occupational stress in the nursing profession has been the focus of much research over the last 20 years (Gray-Toft & Anderson, 1981; Packard & Motowidlo, 1987; Dewe, 1989; Foxall *et al.*, 1990; Tyler & Ellison, 1994; Brown & Edelmann, 2000). However, Dunn and Ritter (1995) have noted that relatively few studies have investigated mental health nurses. Although many of the pressures faced by this group are similar to those reported by staff in other nursing specialities (Riding & Wheeler, 1995), a number of demands relate specifically to mental health settings. These include the often intense nature of nurse–patient interaction (Cronin-Stubbs & Brophy, 1985) and the confrontation of difficult and challenging behaviours on a regular basis (Sullivan, 1993).

Figure 6.2 Structure and organization of elements in a text

ACTIVITY 6.4

Analyse the following texts and decide how these four elements have been organized.

Text 1

The debate surrounding evidence-based practice and the implementation of research-based knowledge in practice is well rehearsed. Some of the key issues discussed have been perceived as barriers to the implementation of knowledge, with Funk *et al.* (1991) developing a 'barriers to research utilization' questionnaire that has been widely adopted in the National Health Service (Retsas 2000; Closs *et al.* 2000; Parahoo 2000). However, these barriers have been mostly framed as individual responsibility – the lack of skill in research critique, the lack of interest in accessing the written knowledge base, the lack of compliance with the evidence (Kaluzny *et al.* 1995; French 1996). (Clarke & Wilcockson 2002, p. 397)

Text 2

While in recent years there has been an increase in the number of studies examining occupational stress among community mental health nurses (Harper & Minghella 1997; McLeod 1997; Coffey 1999; Drake & Brumblecombe 1999; Burnard *et al.* 2000), the experiences of staff in acute inpatient settings, providing 24-hour care for people with serious mental illness, have received less attention. An investigation of acute mental health nursing commissioned for the United Kingdom's (UK) Department of Health (Higgins *et al.* 1997) has highlighted the need for further research in this area. (Jenkins & Elliott 2004, p. 623)

Answers See suggested answers on p. 199.

Table 6.2 presents a checklist of things that you should consider after you have finished writing your argumentative essays. Remember to plan an action to take if your answer to any of the questions has been negative. **As you use the checklist more regularly, add new questions to it so that it becomes more relevant to your needs as a writer.**

The language of arguments

The language of arguments is simple, straightforward and forceful, rather than poetic or fanciful. One of the main linguistic features of argumentative essays is transitional words or connectives (see Chapters 1 and 5). This is because we need to keep arguments either tightly together, as when we want to highlight similarities, or widely apart, as when we want to emphasize how they differ.

Table 6.2 A checklist for the argumentative essay		
Questions	Yes/No	Action if 'no'
1. Have you clearly stated the topic of your argument, its aim(s) and your claims in the **introduction**?		
2. Have you given **reasons** to justify your claims and **support** to your conclusions?		
3. Have you presented a **balanced consideration** of opposing arguments?		
4. Have you used **evidence** to support your claims as well as evidence that supports opposing claims?		
5. Have you briefly **summarized** the claims made, highlighting the main issues or points discussed?		
6. Have you **concluded** in a satisfactory manner, examining implications and making recommendations (if necessary)?		
7.		
8.		

Another common feature of arguments is the use of words that indicate the position of the writers in relation to the argument. This relates to writer stance, as explored in Chapter 3. To indicate this relationship, writers have a set of linguistic tools at their disposal. Some of these are:

- Modal verbs: e.g. 'may', 'can', 'could' to indicate various degrees of possibility; 'would', 'should' and 'will' for various degrees of probability; and 'must', 'have to' and 'ought to' to express degrees of certainty.
- Adverbials: e.g. 'possibly', 'probably', 'certainly'.
- Connectives: e.g. 'in as much as', 'for the reason that', 'consequently'.
- Verbal phrases: e.g. 'it follows that', 'it may be inferred that', 'it may be concluded that'.

What makes argumentative writing 'argumentative'?

One distinguishing feature of argumentative texts is that they go beyond describing or summarizing what has been discussed before. Strong argumentative texts present a critical analysis of existing views, positions and arguments. This critical analysis can be offered to the readers after the evidence supporting an argument has been presented or in the summary section (see 'the structure of argumentation' section above).

At first read, some texts seem to be argumentative. They contain all the elements we have discussed in this unit and their structure and their language are those normally identified with arguments. However, on closer inspection they become just very craftily written descriptions. Consider the following examples:

A)

Strategies for self-care measures, treatment of disease and health care-seeking are related to explanations of disease. According to lay models of illness causation (Helman 2000), illness could be caused by either external or internal factors and by factors related to the individual, nature, social relationships or the supernatural sphere. In the health care-seeking behaviour model (Kleinman 1980), care could be sought in the popular sector (family, friends, relatives), folksector (folk healers; sacred or secular healing) or professional sector (legally sanctioned health care institutions). Health-related behaviour may also be explained by the health belief model (HBM; Rosenstock *et al.* 1988) and perceived locus of control (Rotter 1966). The key components of the HBM are: threat in terms of perceived susceptibility to an ill-health condition (or acceptance of a diagnosis) and perceived seriousness of the condition; outcome expectations expressed as perceived benefits of specified action and perceived barriers to taking that action; and efficacy expectations, that is conviction about one's ability to carry out the recommended action (self-efficacy). Sociodemographic factors such as education, age, sex, race, ethnicity and income are believed to influence behaviour indirectly by affecting these components.

The stronger self-efficacy is perceived to be, the more active and persistent people are. Outcomes interpreted as successful raise self-efficacy. Positive mood enhances perceived self-efficacy, and experiences of mastery have the greatest impact (Bandura 1995).

The general model of locus of control is described in terms of experienced personal control over the environment (Rotter 1966). The model distinguishes between events related to one's own qualities or behaviour (internal locus of control) and circumstances outside one's own control as a result of luck, chance and fate (external locus of control). Those who feel that they have control over their health are more likely to practise health-related behaviour and compliance.

Source: Hjelm, K., P. Nyberg & J. Apelqvist. (2002). Gender influences beliefs about health and illness in diabetic subjects with severe foot lesions. *Journal of Advanced Nursing,* 40(6), 673–84.

B)

In recent years, multiple health risk behaviour research has gained great attention in the academic community (Chung & Joung 2014) and Prochaska has argued that 'multiple health behaviour research represents the future of preventive medicine' (2008, p. 281), an aphorism that can be undeniably applied to nursing and other healthcare professions. This may come as no surprise, for at least four main reasons: First, the high prevalence and the clustering of many health risk behaviours may act synergistically, multiply health consequences and increase the threat to the future health and quality of life in adolescents and young adults (Smpokos *et al.* 2014). Second, evidence suggests that concurrent behaviour change interventions may be more effective when targeting multiple risk factors, e.g. physical inactivity, diet and smoking (Marcus *et al.* 1999; Prochaska & Prochaska 2011; Koniak-Griffin *et al.* 2015). As the resources that can be attributed to public health, health education and health promotion programs are usually limited and, in any case, there is always room for improvement, we need to maximize the effects of our preventive interventions (deRuiter *et al.* 2014). Third, by taking a 'one size fits all' approach, health-promoting interventions may be less successful than programs tailored to individuals or groups (Ferrar *et al.* 2013). McPherson *et al.* (2001), when articulating the homophily principle, argued that people tend to choose people with similar behavioural characteristics. In other words, we need to elucidate, for example, whether individuals who smoke, follow an unhealthy diet and do not exercise at all, share similar characteristics and respond to the same prevention interventions as individuals who only smoke but exercise regularly and eat healthy. Fourth, despite the declining rates in some health risk behaviours (e.g. smoking) and the increasing rates in health-promoting behaviours (e.g. condom use) in certain countries, the interrelationships and co-occurrence among health risk behaviours remain strong (Jackson *et al.* 2012; Hublet *et al.* 2015; Ramiro *et al.* 2015).

Source: Kritsotakis, G., M. Psarrou, M. Vassilaki, Z. Androulaki & A.E. Phi-Lalithis. (2016). Gender differences in the prevalence and clustering of multiple health risk behaviours in young adults. *Journal of Advanced Nursing, 72*(9), 2098–113.

Text A is well organized and well structured in terms of the information it presents to the readers, it uses evidence from academic sources to support its claims, and its language is academic and appropriate. However, it only presents a summary of the existing literature with very little analysis of what the literature means in relation to the topic it refers to. In sum, it is a rather summative and therefore descriptive text that does not convincingly develop its central argument: 'strategies for self-care measures, treatment of disease and health care-seeking are related to explanations of disease', despite its structure, organization, reference to sources and language.

Text B, on the other hand, does not only develop its argument ('multiple health behaviour research represents the future of preventive medicine') in a logical way, using evidence from sources, but it does so in a persuasive way. It structures the main reasons supporting the central argument by using logical connectives (e.g. 'First', 'second') (see also Chapter 8), and adds a critical analysis of the main reasons which are supported by the right use of argumentative language (e.g. 'This means', 'in other words'). Equally importantly, after presenting, supporting and analysing each main idea in the argument, the text calls for an action to be taken (e.g. 'we need to maximize the effects'), creating a sense of involvement for the readers and raising their awareness of the importance of the main ideas and issues at the same time.

As you can see, Text B presents a clear organization of ideas (followed by supporting evidence and critical analysis), a logically developed and very effective structure (mainly achieved by the use of logical connectives), and a powerful and convincing way of involving the readers by calling them to action.

ACTIVITY 6.5

Read these two versions of the same text: Version 1 is merely descriptive and Version 2 is argumentative. Underline those features of language that have helped to make the second version argumentative.

Version 1

The differences seen are not explainable by disappointment with the care-giver assignment. Staniszewska and Ahmed (1999) point out that patients' expectations are influenced by their awareness of what they realistically expect. Evaluation of a service is also influenced by beliefs about the duty the service owes the client and whether or not there were circumstances outside the service's control that affected the care (Williams *et al.* 1998). If expectations are a determinant of satisfaction with care, there is then less difference between the satisfaction scores of the two groups since women have different expectations for doctors than they do for midwives. (Adapted from Harvey *et al.* 2002, p. 266)

Version 2

It is possible, however, that the differences seen are not entirely explainable by disappointment with the care-giver assignment. Staniszewska and Ahmed (1999) point out that patients' expectations are influenced by their awareness of what they might realistically expect. Evaluation of a service is also influenced by beliefs about the duty the service owes the client and whether or not there were circumstances outside the service's control that affected the care (Williams *et al.* 1998). If expectations are a determinant of satisfaction with care, it is possible that there would have been less difference between the satisfaction scores of the two groups since women have different expectations for doctors than they do for midwives. (Harvey *et al.* 2002, p. 266)

Answers See suggested answers on p. 200.

Grammar and English use

In this last section of the chapter, you will find some suggestions about how to deal with grammar and language-use problems that many students experience when writing argumentative texts. More specifically, this section deals with the language of argumentation. If you need more detail on any of these topics, see the Glossary of Key Terms and the list of Further Readings and Resources at the end of the book.

Modal verbs

Modal verbs are special verbs that indicate 'the way or mode' in which something is done or said. In sentence (1) the modal verb 'will' does not indicate the future but the way in which the speaker sees the possibility of something happening. In sentence (2) the speaker appears less certain and therefore chooses to decrease the level of certainty by using 'may'.

(1)   The patient **will** find it difficult to adjust herself to her new lifestyle.
(2)   The patient **may** find it difficult to adjust herself to her new lifestyle.

Table 6.3 shows you the most frequent uses of common modal verbs, followed by some examples.

Table 6.3 The use of modal verbs		
Modal verb	**Meaning 1**	**Meaning 2**
Can	*Ability* She **can** speak many languages, which has helped her deal with her diverse patients.	*Possibility* (1) The results of this study **can** make a real impact on the professional practice of midwives.
Could	*Possibility* (2) You **could** spend the rest of your free time revising for your exams tomorrow.	*Suggestion* These results **could** indicate that progress can be a slippery concept.
Have to	*Certainty* (1) That **has to** be the right dose for a patient in his condition.	*Obligation* (1) You **have to** follow the doctor's orders if you want to be discharged from hospital soon.

Modal verb	Meaning 1	Meaning 2
May	*Possibility* (3) Under his psychiatric conditions, the patient **may** temporarily lose control over his or her actions.	*Permission* Patients **may** not bring their own personal belongings with them unless they are told to do so.
Might	*Possibility* (4) Under his psychiatric conditions, the patient **might** temporarily lose control over his or her actions.	*Suggestion* You **might** not want to be alone when you come to collect the results of the test.
Must	*Certainty* (2) That **must** have been the best possible way of doing it.	*Obligation* (2) You **must** bring with you a proof of identity and your medical record number.
Shall	*Inevitability* The drug **shall** react in a matter of seconds.	*Promise* I **shall** make the shift arrangements for tomorrow.
Should	*Recommendation* They **should** have followed the directions as they were indicated.	*Assumption* They **should** be here by now.

As you can see from Table 6.3, there are various possibilities to express a similar meaning, indicated by the numbers between brackets. For example, there are at least four different ways of expressing possibility. These ways can be put on a cline to indicate different degrees, as indicated in Figure 6.3.

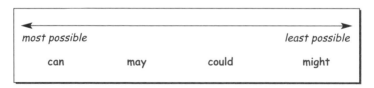

Figure 6.3 **Degrees of possibility**

Simply put, the difference in meaning among sentences (3) to (6) is only one of the degree of possibility.

(3) The results of this study **can** make a real impact on the professional practice of midwives.

(4) The results of this study **may** make a real impact on the professional practice of midwives.

(5) The results of this study **could** make a real impact on the professional practice of midwives.

(6) The results of this study **might** make a real impact on the professional practice of midwives.

Adverbials

Adverbials can also be used to indicate the writer's stance in relation to the claims made. Again, we could say that the difference between sentences (7) and (8) is one of degree.

(7) The patient has made a speedy recovery.

(8) The patient has **certainly** made a speedy recovery.

Other adverbials that indicate the writer's stance include possibly, probably, certainly, definitely, inevitably, forcefully, successfully, unfortunately.

Verbal phrases

Verbal phrases that contain verbs such as 'seem', 'appear' or 'look', and phrasal verbs or adverbials like the ones described above, can also be used to indicate stance. Sentences (9) to (11) show not only the degree of certainty of the writer, but also the writer's stance in term of the claims being made.

(9)   Considering the results, **it may be concluded that** the tests have failed.

(10) Considering the results, **it seems that** the tests have failed.

(11) Considering the results, the tests **have failed**.

Revising the objectives of this chapter

Tick those objectives that you feel you have achieved and review those you have not yet managed to accomplish. Then, complete the **Achievement Chart** at the back of the book.

In this chapter, you have learnt to:

☐ recognize the difference between opinion and argumentation

☐ identify the strength of an argument

☐ structure arguments effectively

☐ identify the main language items used in argumentative writing.

How to Write in Other Genres

At the end of this chapter, you should be able to:

- write action plans
- write care plans
- prepare, write and choose an appropriate format for portfolios, including e-portfolios
- use a personal diary template
- produce reports
- write systematic reviews
- respond to case studies
- identify effective ways of producing dissertation proposals
- plan to start writing your dissertation.

Other common genres

In this chapter you will explore other common genres in nursing and midwifery: action and care plans, portfolios, personal diaries, reports, systematic reviews, case studies for assessment purposes, and research proposals.

The chapter opens with an examination of what action plans are and what information you will need to complete them. It then moves on to describe care plans and examines the type of information and language that you use to complete them. Next, you will analyse portfolios. The section on portfolios provides you with a fairly comprehensive coverage of the topic: what portfolios and e-portfolios are, what they contain, how they can be formatted and how they are normally assessed.

The last part of the chapter deals with personal diaries, reports, systematic reviews, case studies for assessment purposes, and the research proposal. In the research proposal section, you will find information about how to prepare and present a proposal, together with tips on what to include in each section and the appropriate style to use. Finally, you will discover tips on how to get organized to write your undergraduate dissertation.

How to write action plans

Students often ask whether action plans are the same as 'to-do' lists. These do share some similarities, but they are not the same. To-do lists enumerate all the tasks that you need to carry out. They are useful reminders of what you have to do. They can include a priority ranking: you can rank each of the tasks as 'high priority', 'medium priority' or 'low priority'. Table 7.1 shows you what a to-do list looks like.

Table 7.1 A to-do list with priority ranking	
Task	Priority (H = High, M = Medium, L = Low)
1. Read Chapters 5 & 6 in Atkinson's book for exam.	H
2. Return books to library before end of next week.	M
3. Email John & Marcia about a get-together after exams.	L

Action plans, in contrast, do not only lay out the task you will concentrate on, they also include a detailed description of the steps to be taken to perform the task successfully. Action plans also include challenges that you might face in carrying out the tasks, and strategies that you can use to deal with them. It is also important that you give the task at hand a deadline for completion.

The information you enter in an action plan will help you monitor and assess your progress and record any changes that have been made in the process of getting things done. Action plans can be used on their own or they can be part of other documents such as your personal development plan or your portfolio (see later in this chapter). Table 7.2 illustrates an action plan for a very simple task: read two book chapters as preparation for an exam. Although you may not need a detailed action plan for simple tasks like this one, it is always a good idea to start with laying out simple tasks. As you get more practice, you will see that you don't need so many details and that your language in describing tasks, challenges and strategies becomes simpler and simpler.

The language and style of action plans are simple and straightforward. As illustrated in Table 7.2, you don't need to use complete sentences, as notes will do. You will need different tenses for the different sections of an action plan. Infinitives or the simple present tense are used to provide a short description of the task, the simple future to describe challenges and strategies, the present perfect tense to record progress and the simple past to indicate the completion of the task, though a simple date indicating when the task was completed would do.

Table 7.2 Action plan for exam preparation

Task	Steps	Challenges (CH)/Strategies (ST)	Progress	Completion
1. Read Chapter 5 (Atkinson) for exam in 2 wks.	1.1 Borrow book from library.	May not find available copy at library. (CH) Will have to borrow copy from another student & photocopy. (ST) Who will you call?	Done – there was a copy in library	Day 1
	1.2 Read Chapter 5 through.	Interruptions by flatmates. (CH) Study at library. (ST)	Finished reading	Day 1
	1.3 Underline main ideas.	May not find them easily. (CH) Photocopy & colour-code. (ST)	Done	Day 1
	1.4 Summarize main ideas.	Put ideas coded in same colour together. (ST)	Done	Day 1
	1.5 Read and write summary in own words.	Difficult to paraphrase, find synonymous expressions. (CH) Use dictionary/thesaurus. (ST)	Will do tomorrow/done on day 2	Day 2
2. Read Chapter 6 (Atkinson) for exam in 2 wks.	2.1 Read Chapter 6 through.	Interruptions by flatmates. (CH) Study at library. (ST)	Finished reading	Day 2
	2.2 Underline main ideas.	May not find them easily. (CH) Photocopy & colour-code. (ST)	Done	Day 2
	2.3 Summarize main ideas.	Put ideas coded in same colour together. (ST)	Done	Day 2
	2.4 Read and write summary in own words.	Difficult to paraphrase, find synonymous expressions. (CH) Use dictionary/thesaurus. (ST)	Done	Day 2

How to write care plans

What are care plans? Care plans are documents that provide a detailed description of the plan of care to be provided to a patient. Traditionally, care plans have been regarded as the sole domain of nurses, but with the increase in the involvement of interdisciplinary teams in the care of patients this should no longer be the case. In fact, for care plans to be effective, their design and implementation should engage not only nurses, but all the professionals who are involved in providing the care to the patient.

Care plan documents will normally include:

- The patient's name, his/her medical record number and his/her room number.
- Date and description of the patient's needs and problems.
- Nursing diagnoses (though this will depend on your work setting).
- Goal setting.
- Interventions needed to achieve the goals.
- Assessment of progress.
- Re-evaluation of care plan.

What steps are followed in designing care plans? Your work setting may have an established protocol for care plans or may only have general guidelines, but most care plans will start by evaluating the patient's needs. This is referred to as the **first step**, and normally involves assessing the patient on admission.

The **second step** requires a problem list to be drawn up. Again, depending on your work setting, this may simply mean a list of medical diagnoses, but it could involve more complicated protocols.

The **third step** is closely related to the second. Here you use information that comes from asking questions such as 'How can this be solved/improved?' for each of the problems on your list, followed by setting a goal to improve the problem. It is important to remember that each of the goals that you set should be SMART (Specific, Measurable, Attainable, Realistic and Time-oriented).

The **fourth step** will describe the actions or interventions needed to achieve each goal. The **fifth step** assesses the progress made by the patient and re-evaluates the care plan to adjust it to the patient's changed needs. Figure 7.1 shows you the relationship of the five steps.

How are care plans written? What language is used and what tenses are required? The different parts of the care plan will require different language and tenses.

- **Description of problem/need**: Give a general label to the problem (e.g. communication), followed by a short description (e.g. has difficulty understanding what is being said). This is mainly expressed in a present tense (the present perfect may also be used). You don't normally need subjects and there is a tendency not to use articles ('the', 'a' etc.). For example, (*patient*) **has** (simple present) *knowledge deficit regarding transmission, complications and treatment of Chlamydia*, or *patient* **has been diagnosed** (present perfect) *with breast cancer.*

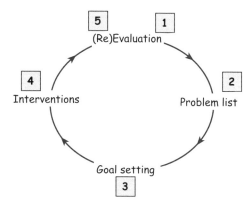

Figure 7.1 Steps in care planning

- **Goal setting**: state the goal in simple terms, followed by the deadline expressed in days or months (use 'will' and verbal phrases such as 'be able to') as, for example, *resident with a stroke* **will** *be able to communicate his basic needs in two months.* Avoid expressing two or more goals together. This would make it difficult for you to evaluate progress on each. The patient may make good progress towards one goal but not the other.
- **Approach planning**: state actions/interventions in simple terms. Use verbs in their base form. For example, **use** (a base form of a verb) *plain, simple, concrete language when speaking with resident.*
- **Re-evaluation**: express results of the re-evaluation of care in simple terms, by saying what happened. Use the present perfect tense for this. For example, *patient* **has learnt** (present perfect) *to express his basic needs in simple but clear language.* If the re-evaluation shows that you need to set new goals, use the same language and tenses as in goal setting above. For example, *patient has a knowledge deficit regarding the transmission, complications and treatment of Chlamydia,* or *patient has been diagnosed with breast cancer.*

ACTIVITY 7.1

Here is a short summary of the situation of Mrs M. Read it and fill in the care plan below. Complete as much as you can and then check with the suggested answer at the end of the book.

Mrs M, 65, has been hospitalized for the second time this month. Her medical record number is ICD-9-CM 348.1 and she is in room 231. She presents a severe loss of self-image and self-esteem due to effects of chemotherapy.

Patient's name		
Medical record number		
Room number		
Date		
Problem	Description	Goal
Approach	Assessment	Review (re-evaluation)

Answers See suggested answers on p. 200.

How to write portfolios

This section of the chapter examines portfolios as a tool for academic and professional development.

A student portfolio may be defined as a tool to:

- Assess a student's performance in a comprehensive manner.
- Study the work done by a student.
- Identify strengths and weaknesses in the learning path taken by a student.
- Analyse recent achievements.
- Decide on a course of action to ensure development.

A professional portfolio is also a very important tool in the nursing and midwifery professions. A professional portfolio is a collection of documents that give evidence of a person's professional career.

These documents can be used as the basis for a person's

- curriculum vitae;
- career path;
- promotion;
- continuous professional development.

Portfolios contain a collection of a student's or a professional's work over a period of time. These pieces of work are used as evidence of academic or professional development, achievement and needs.

The contents of a portfolio will obviously vary depending on whether it is a student or a professional portfolio. The student portfolio will normally contain:

- **A statement of purpose:** the main reasons you are writing this portfolio.
- **Personal information:** name, contact details, other relevant ID.
- **Clinical experience:** clinical placements, work experience (including assignments you have written on this).
- **Assignments:** a selection of assignments that show the academic progress you have made so far.
- **Reflective documents:** a reflective essay (see Chapter 4) critically showing how you have developed since you started your course or your university programme, and your personal development planning – where you have been, where you are, where you would like to be and how you will get there (skills and knowledge needed).
- **Personal development plans** and **action plans.**

The professional portfolio will contain:

- **A statement of purpose:** the main reasons you are writing this portfolio.
- **Personal information:** name, contact details, registration details, other relevant ID.
- **Education:** schools, colleges and universities you have previously attended, courses you have taken, other relevant information (including copies of certificates, examination results, transcripts etc.), other professional qualifications.
- **Record of employment:** professional posts within the discipline, professional posts outside the discipline (including copies of job descriptions or brief description of duties and responsibilities).
- **Professional development:** clinical supervision, research and project work, conferences and seminars participated in and attended, memberships of professional bodies (including details), personal development plans.
- **Reflective documents:** a reflective piece of writing critically showing how you have developed since you started your career, and your personal development planning – where you have been, where you are, where you would like to be and how you will get there (skills and knowledge needed), as well as action plans.

As you can see, reflective writing is the central document in both kinds of portfolios. In this piece of writing, students and professionals can use their critical skills to reflect on their strengths and weaknesses, to plan their personal growth and to decide on a course of action to pursue their professional development.

> **Glossary**
> Critical skills

In 2005 the NHS (National Health Service) in the United Kingdom set up an e-portfolio platform to support health professionals' achievement, reflection and learning. This platform can be found at www.nhseportfolios.org/Anon/Login/Login.aspx. (Last accessed on 23 March 2018.)

A portfolio can be either paper-based or electronic. Both have advantages and disadvantages. Paper-based portfolios are easy to handle and display, and are self-contained products. However, they are also less flexible, less appropriate for documents of various sizes, and more difficult to expand over a long period. Electronic portfolios are very flexible and easy to expand, can incorporate documents of almost any size and in any format (e.g. video clips, audio files), but they are dependent on a computer for display. This means that arrangements have to be made in advance to view the portfolio.

Paper-based portfolios can be stored and presented in:

- ring binders or folders;
- plastic ringers;
- plastic folders;
- tab dividers.

Electronic portfolios (also called e-portfolios, digital or online portfolios) can be stored and presented in:

- memory sticks or cards;
- CDs;
- DVDs.

An e-portfolio may include:

- Text or writing samples;
- Electronic files;
- Images and or audio files;
- Multimedia content;
- Videos;
- PowerPoint presentations;
- Blog entries, and
- Hyperlinks.

Free access examples of e-portfolios for a variety of purposes can be seen on the following websites (all websites last accessed on 23 March 2018):

- http://wp.auburn.edu/writing/eportfolio-project/eportfolio-examples/
- www.youtube.com/watch?v=6B3tujXlbdk
- https://uwaterloo.ca/centre-for-teaching-excellence/resources/integrative-learning/eport-folios/examples-student-eportfolios
- www.digication.com
- https://mahara.org

Finally, let us have a look at some of the criteria commonly used to assess portfolios. Portfolios are normally assessed in three areas:

- **Organization**: Has the content been logically organized? Do the documents in each section reflect the aims and objectives of the section?
- **Content**: Have the documents been appropriately chosen? Do the documents represent strong evidence of the portfolio owner's knowledge and skills? Does the quality of the documents offer evidence of the owner's skills and values?
- **Presentation**: Are the entries well written? Do they demonstrate problems with spelling and grammar? Does the portfolio look professional? Does it create a positive image of the owner?

Keeping a personal diary

A personal diary is a written account used to record, reflect on and sometimes assess the experiences, progress and achievements of the owner in areas as diverse as cognitive, study and communication skills, learning responsibility and independence, reflective skills, improving practice and professional development. A personal diary can also be used as written evidence of all of this, and can thus be linked to the owner's own portfolio (see how to write portfolios earlier in the chapter).

There are many types of personal diaries and all will have their own distinctive features, but most will allow the owner to:

- Organize the records in a given way (chronologically, thematically etc.).
- Jot down both brief descriptive as well as reflective notes.
- Control the content and style.
- Record experiences on an incremental basis (over a period of time).

The template in Table 7.3 is merely an indication of what a personal diary may look like. In this particular case, the template allows users to give each experience they want to record a short label (e.g. improving practice) that they can later use to retrieve it more easily, especially when there are many entries in their diary. It also offers them the opportunity to record what their feelings and thoughts were at the moment of the experience and to revisit these at a later stage. Next, the template allows users to identify the key issues on which they need to reflect, which may happen right after the experience and sometimes later on. Finally, the template also provides space for noting down what the user has learnt from the experience, how their learning took place, and what they need to do next to complete their learning experience.

It is advisable to try to decide which reflective model you want to use quite early. For example, you may wish to use Gibbs' model (1988) or Driscoll's (1994). If you have no or little previous experience in using diaries, you may perhaps want to start with this template, which has been largely designed following Gibbs'

Table 7.3 A personal diary template

Experience (use a 'label' that can help you identify this experience easily)	Date	What happened (brief description)	Thoughts & feelings	Relevant issues (to reflect on)	Learning		
					What?	How?	What next?

model of reflection. However, as you become more familiar with keeping a personal diary and depending on your reasons for keeping it, it will be a better idea for you to develop your own diary style. Your decision about how to structure your diary will depend on factors such as your learning and writing styles, how you best reflect on your experiences, and how you achieve your objectives.

How to write reports

You will be asked to write reports as a student and later on as a professional. Simply defined, reports are documents that:

- Have a very clear objective and a specific purpose.
- Are written for a specific audience.
- Have a distinctive structure and layout.
- Contain information as well as recommendations.

As you can see, reports are distinctive documents and as such they differ from other genres that we have covered before. A report does not discuss opinions or theories, but presents and analyses information, and makes recommendations on which the reader is expected to act.

There are different types of reports, which can be put on a cline going from the *academic report* on one end to the *professional report* on the other. Figure 7.2 shows such a cline.

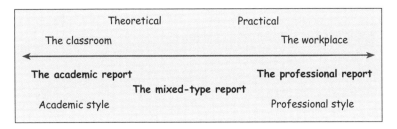

Figure 7.2 **The report type cline**

Reports are written for different purposes and with different audiences in mind. Both the purpose and the audience of a report will determine its content as well as its structure. Lecturers, for example, ask students to write reports as assignments. These will be *academic reports*. As shown in Figure 7.2, the academic report is more theoretical in nature and will observe all the academic conventions that you have analysed in the previous chapters of this book. The report that students may be asked to write after a work placement is an example of an academic report. It is a formal piece of writing, focusing on the theoretical aspects of an issue, and its recommendations will result from an analysis of the literature used in preparation for the report. You will be most probably asked to use your placement experience to illustrate the theoretical points you are reporting, but the focus will still be on theory.

The *professional report*, on the other hand, tends to be more practical in nature and aims at solving a given problem or situation. Its recommendations or evaluations will then be oriented to solving the problem or improving the situation being analysed. Professional reports normally follow the style of the workplace for which they have been written. In the health-care sector in the UK there are many types of reports produced for and by the NHS. There are, for instance, investigation reports that examine the causes of serious problems in the provision of good-quality care to its patients. The main aim here is to make recommendations to solve the problems under investigation. Another example of professional reports is the staff survey report that gathers information to help improve the working lives of care providers within the organization.

Mixed-type reports result from situations where there is a combination of writers, purposes or audiences. For example, a business person who normally writes professional reports may be asked to write a report as an example to be used in a business class. In this case, the purpose of the report – a pedagogical purpose – will require the writer to produce a mixed-type report. Similarly, a university student on a work placement, who normally writes academic reports, may be asked to produce a report for the company where s/he is on placement. In this case the writer is a student but s/he will be writing for a professional audience. This again will produce a mixed-type report.

How are reports structured? Consider the following three principles that will give shape to your reports:

- audience;
- aim(s) and purpose(s);
- contents.

So the questions you need to ask at the planning stage are:

- **Who** am I writing this for? What do they know about this? What do they want to do with this report?
- **Why** am I writing this?
- **What** will the reader need to know to make informed decisions?

These three elements are closely interrelated, and each will influence the others. Thus, if your report is:

- expected to **encourage further thinking** about the issue(s) it examines, then its **findings section** is the most crucial.
- an account of something you have **observed**, then its **recommendations section** is the most vital.

- on an in-progress **project**, then the sections where it deals with the **evidence** and makes its **recommendations** are critical.

Once you have answered these questions and considered how they are related, it is time for you to decide on the different parts of the report. This section will focus on *academic reports*, as they will be the most frequently required in your academic life. There are three main sections that your academic reports should have: the **preliminaries**, the **body** and the **end matter**. The list below shows you the different components of each of these sections, followed by a more detailed discussion of the essential ones.

Preliminaries

- *Cover sheet* (title of report, your name, the name of the institution, the date you produced the report).
- *Title page* (full title of report, your name).
- *Acknowledgements* (acknowledge the people who have helped or supported you).
- *Table of contents* (list different sections together with their page number).
- *Abstract/Summary/Executive summary* (an abstract of the complete report: the procedure followed, initial findings, conclusions and recommendations).

Body

- *Aims and purposes* (why you wrote the report).
- *Literature review* (critical analysis of the literature related to your report).
- *Methodology* (type of methods used, data collection and ethical issues).
- *Results* (what you found out, using graphs, tables and figures to support text).
- *Analysis* (critical interpretation of results).
- *Conclusions* (the conclusions you arrived at).
- *Recommendations* (what course of action should be taken considering your conclusions).

End matter

- *References* (sources cited in your report).
- *Bibliography* (sources you consulted but did not cite).
- *Appendices* (supporting evidence/graphs/statistics etc. that are too long to be included in the body).

Let's consider the most essential components of each of these parts. Obviously, the central element in the preliminaries is the *abstract*. The abstract of a report should summarize:

- The **problem** investigated.
- The **action** taken to investigate the problem.
- The **results** from such an action.

One thing you should keep in mind about the abstract is that it is not a kind of introduction but a summary of the whole report, so don't get tempted to repeat the contents of your introduction here. Your abstract should be concise – no more than 200 words – and informative at the same time, and it should summarize the points mentioned above.

The components of the body of a report are all important. However, some are more relevant than others, depending on what is reported. The methodology and presentation of the results, for instance, are more relevant to reports on experimental research than to those on reviews of the existing literature. While a report can refer to the methodology of a given study or experiment, it may be more difficult to describe and examine the different methods used in different studies in the relevant literature.

This section will analyse those components of the body that are relevant to reports on experiments as well as a review of the literature. They are:

- *Literature review*
- *Analysis of results*
- *Conclusions*
- *Recommendations*

ACTIVITY 7.2

These two texts come from the same report. Compare them and decide which is (i) part of the abstract; (ii) part of the introduction of the report.

Text 1

Although simulation as a pedagogical tool has been used in many university programmes, it has been more widely implemented in business and medical degree programmes (Hook 2003; Morton & Rauen 2004; Robinson 2001). In nursing, simulation has been investigated for more than 20 years now, especially in the US academic context. Simulation has been identified as a pedagogical tool that can help nursing students operate in a 'microworld' in which their actions and interactions can be studied, explored and used for training purposes (Gordon & Cooper 2004). Patient simulators, for example, give nursing students all the information they need to make clinical decisions.

Text 2

The pedagogical value of simulation in university programmes has been under investigation for the last 30 years. The Nursing and Midwifery Council (NMC) in the UK has now started a pilot programme to investigate the benefits of using simulation to help nursing students to be fit for practice before registration. This report presents the results of researching the previous applications of simulation in various other university degree programmes, examining the results from such applications, and analysing the pedagogical and professional implications of applying simulation in degree programmes. Based on these considerations, the report makes recommendations as to what approaches to implementing simulation in nursing should be followed.

Answers See suggested answers on p. 200.

The key section in the body is the literature review. The rest of the sections will be based on the issues discussed in this component. As stated above, the literature review presents a critical analysis (not a summary!) of major works in the field or topic of the report (see also later in this chapter).

The analysis of the results is another important part of the body of a report. Here you will have to examine the importance and relevance of the results presented in the studies that you reviewed in the literature. You will also have to refer to the implications of the results for the issues about which you are writing.

The next section presents what you can conclude based on the evidence found in the literature review and the analysis of results. It is important here to follow the logical principles you examined in relation to writing an argument in Chapter 6. A conclusion is only relevant to a discussion as long as it results from the evidence presented and analysed in that discussion. This is especially important when you have to make recommendations, as they will be based on your conclusions.

Thus recommendations should establish a logical link between the different issues discussed in the body of the report and the conclusions that you arrived at after analysing the results. The same principles apply here as those about making sensible recommendations that you examined in relation to the care critique in Chapter 5. Reproduced on the following page as Figure 7.3 is the relationship between issues, conclusion and recommendations.

In the 'end matter', the last section of a report, the main component is its list of references. As you may remember from Chapter 1, a list of references should contain only those sources mentioned in the body of the text (see also Chapter 10). A bibliography list is also important as it may be used to direct the reader to sources of information that you consulted for the preparation of the report. Although these sources have not been cited in the body of the report, they can serve as further references to the reader.

Figure 7.3 The relationship between conclusion and recommendations

Finally, here are some notes on the style of reports. Remember to observe conventions for referencing and for presenting your final product. If necessary, please refer to Chapters 1 (conventions) and 10 (referencing).

- Unlike essays, reports do not always use continuous prose. What is more, most reports will combine some prose in the form of short paragraphs with bullet points, something that is avoided in essay writing.
- Most reports will have numbered headings and subheadings to guide the reader through their contents and to make it easier for them to find specific information more quickly and effectively.
- Reports will also contain a considerable number of tables, charts and graphs.

Before writing your report, it would be very useful for you to visit the websites of some multinational corporations and download their annual reports to see some good examples. You can access company reports by clicking on 'about us/name of company' or 'company', and then on 'corporate information' or 'investors'. Alternatively, you can consult some of the resources for using tables, charts and graphs listed at the end of this book.

How to write systematic reviews

What is a systematic review?
A systematic review is a rigorous evaluation of evidence from research studies and other documents based on a peer-reviewed protocol. It can examine quantitative or qualitative evidence or a mix of both. Systematic reviews that examine both qualitative and quantitative evidence are called mixed-method systematic reviews.
A systematic review aims to

- **identify** published and unpublished evidence relevant to a well-defined health-care question;
- **select** evidence to be incorporated in the review based on a specific set of inclusion/exclusion criteria (also called 'the review protocol');

- **evaluate** the quality of the evidence included;
- **synthesize** the findings and contributions made by the evidence;
- **interpret** critically such findings in the light of the health-care question; and
- **present** a balanced (strengths and weaknesses) and impartial summary of the findings in terms of how appropriate and meaningful they are.

Glossary
Appropriate
Meaningful
Rigorous
Synthesize

Seven steps to writing a systematic review

1   *Determining the need for a new systematic review*

Before you start working on your systematic review, it is advisable that you check whether a review on the health-care question you want to investigate has been carried out already. This will help you decide whether your review is needed or you need to modify or change your question. To determine the need for your systematic review, you could begin by searching databases and reliable websites such as the:

- ANZCA: Australian health and education databases and websites (Australia): www.anzca.edu.au/resources/library/databases
- Campbell Library of Systematic Reviews (Norway): www.campbellcollaboration.org/library.php
- Cochrane Database of Systematic Reviews (UK): www.cochranelibrary.com/about/about-cochrane-systematic-reviews.html
- Database of Abstracts of Reviews of Effects (UK): http://community.cochrane.org/editorial-and-publishing-policy-resource/ overview-cochrane-library-and-related-content/databases-included-cochrane- library/database-abstracts-reviews-effects-dare
- Evidence for Policy and Practice Information (UK): https://eppi.ioe.ac.uk/cms/Default.aspx?tabid=185
- HealthData.gov (USA): www.healthdata.gov
- Health Services Research Information Central (HSRIC, USA): www.nlm.nih.gov/hsrinfo/datasites.html#164Databases/Repositories
- MEDLINE (USA): www.nlm.nih.gov/bsd/pmresources.html
- National Community Mental Health Care Database (Australia): www.aihw.gov.au/about-our-data
- National Institute for Health and Care Excellence (NICE, UK): www.nice.org.uk

- NZ health statistics (New Zealand):
  www.health.govt.nz/nz-health-statistics
- Systematic Review Data Repository (SRDR, USA):
  https://srdr.ahrq.gov

(All websites last accessed on 23 March 2018)

Searching databases and websites such as these serves two main purposes. First, it will help you determine what has been done in the area of your health-care question before you decide to go ahead with your systematic review. Second, it will guide you into deciding what evidence you could use for your own review (see 4 and 5 below).

2 Defining an appropriate health-care question

The health-care question (or questions if there is more than one) that your systematic review will investigate is the most important starting point for your investigation. Together with the design of the methodology it will form the basis for the inclusion criteria used for selecting the evidence (the review protocol). The question can be framed in terms of the:

- participants;
- interventions;
- design; and
- outcomes of the evidence to be included in the review.

Once you are satisfied with the question or questions your systematic review will investigate, it is a good idea to seek feedback from a number of people. For example, you can start with other students in your group, then seek your supervisor's feedback, and finally use stakeholder input (e.g. patients, health-care institutions, professional associations) to refine your question(s).

Take a look at systematic reviews that have been published in your area of investigation to see how questions have been formulated. For instance, King & Flenady (2002) conducted a systematic review to 'assess the effects of prophylactic antibiotics on preterm labour'. To achieve this objective they formulated their question in the following way: 'Since rupture of the membranes is an important factor in the progression of preterm labour, it is important to see if the routine administration of antibiotics confers any benefit or causes harm, prior to membrane rupture.' (Note that questions do not always need to include question marks.)

In another work, McDaid and colleagues (2005) did a review to evaluate 'the clinical effectiveness of treatments for childhood retinoblastoma'. Their review included studies that investigated **participants** diagnosed with retinoblastoma at the age of 18 or under that had followed them into adulthood. These studies reported a combination of **interventions**, including enucleation, external beam radiotherapy, thermotherapy and photocoagulation. In terms of the **design**, the studies included in their review favoured randomized controlled trials (RCTs) although cohort studies were also eligible. Finally, the outcomes considered included: survival, tumour response, visual acuity and disease remission.

3 *Building the review protocol*

The review protocol sets out the methods to be used and the processes to be followed for the review. It should include the:

- **background** (why the review is needed, the rationale for the inclusion criteria, and the focus of the question or questions);
- **question** or questions to be reviewed (stated clearly and precisely);
- **inclusion criteria** (what evidence will be included in relation to the population, interventions, design, and outcomes of the evidence stated in the question or questions);
- **search strategy**, including what databases and websites will be consulted;
- **study selection**;
- **quality assessment** (see section 4 below); and
- **data synthesis**.

Building the protocol in advance and adhering to it reduces the risk of introducing bias to the review (e.g. selecting only studies that support the review questions). Bias may also result from considering evidence published only in a particular language (e.g. English). Therefore, serious consideration should be given to whether studies in different languages (e.g. languages other than English) will be included or excluded from the review, together with a rationale for this choice.

Similarly, an unbiased and comprehensive systematic review will consider evidence published not only in peer-reviewed journals, but also in materials not formally published such as reports, book chapters, conference abstracts and proceedings, and theses. These are usually called 'grey literature'.

4 *Searching the literature for evidence*

As shown in section 1, there are a number of sources that should be consulted. It is important to use a 'standardized search filter' to find the right evidence in the databases and websites. A standardized search filter is a strategy (e.g. key words) that you design to retrieve valid studies from the literature. A filter will help you identify particular publications most likely to answer a health-care question you want to investigate.

Grey literature can be searched by using search engines and websites too. Similarly, expert opinion can be sought by contacting key authors for expansion or clarification.

As you have probably realized by now, not all evidence is regarded as being of the same quality. It is important, therefore, that you familiarize yourself with the quality of the evidence you plan to include in your review. The quality of your review will depend on the quality of the evidence it includes. There is a 'hierarchy of evidence' whose quality goes from strongest (randomized controlled trials) to weakest (expert opinion):

- **Randomized controlled trials** (RCT), including randomized cross-over trials and cluster randomized trials
- **Quasi-experimental studies**, including non-randomized controlled studies, before-and-after studies, interrupted time series
- **Observational studies**, including cohort studies, case-control studies, and case series
- **Expert opinion.**

5 *Assessing the evidence*

Once you have finished searching the literature for evidence, you need to assess each piece of evidence (e.g. journal article, report, working paper). The assessment criteria should include:

- **eligibility**, following the inclusion criteria;
- **quality and appropriateness of the methodology** used; and
- **reported findings.**

The assessment of each piece of evidence should ideally be conducted by two reviewers independently. If another student in your course is working on a similar health-care area, you could be each other's independent reviewer.

Finally, make **a list of the studies that will be included** in your systematic review (those that have met the inclusion criteria), and a list of those you have excluded with a clear rationale for this decision.

6 *Synthesizing the findings*

You should synthesize the findings from the studies that you have included in your review. Synthesizing findings means organizing the information the studies provide around the specific question or questions that your systematic review has investigated.

For example, if the review aims to 'improve conceptual clarity of interprofessional interventions' (Reeves *et al.* 2010), the findings should be synthesized around issues such as:

- approaches to conceptualization, implementation, and assessment of interprofessional interventions;
- types of interprofessional interventions: for instance, interprofessional education; interprofessional practice; and interprofessional organization; and
- the nature of each type of intervention by stage, participants, interprofessional objectives, and outcomes.

If your review has included qualitative evidence, then the review will present a **meta-synthesis** of the results. A meta-synthesis is a systematic integration of results from a number of different but interrelated qualitative studies.

If it has included quantitative evidence, the review will present a **meta-analysis** of the results. A meta-analysis is a statistical analysis that examines the findings of multiple, homogeneous empirical studies. The main aim of a meta-analysis is to achieve a higher statistical power and more robust conclusions than would be possible from analysing only one study.

7 *Presenting a balanced and impartial summary*

The results from synthesizing the findings need to be discussed in the context of your health-care question or questions. This should include the quality of the studies that were selected and the contributions they have made to the area of your research. Finally, the applicability of the findings to the context explored by the health-care question should also be discussed.

Checklist for assessing systematic reviews

This checklist can be used to assess the quality of your review once you finish writing the first draft. It can also be used to evaluate the quality of the studies that you have found before deciding whether to include them in your review (Table 7.4).

Table 7.4 Checklist for assessing systematic reviews		
Area	Key question	Sub-question(s)
Topic	Is the topic worth investigating?	Does it cover areas not previously investigated thoroughly?
	If so, is it well defined?	Does it include the population, interventions, design, and outcomes?
Evidence search	Was the search for evidence thorough?	Was the search strategy defined? Was 'grey literature' considered? Were non-English language publications considered? If not, was a rationale for not considering them presented?
Inclusion criteria	Were the inclusion criteria described?	Were details of study selection and eligibility criteria provided? Were inclusion and exclusion rationales given?
Quality	How was the quality of the evidence included assessed?	Were the outcomes assessed by their robustness? How was bias controlled? Was additional information from the authors sought?
Chance effect	Was the possibility of outcomes having occurred by chance assessed?	How was it controlled?
Recommendations	Were the recommendations based on the quality of the evidence?	How strong was the relationship between the evidence and the recommendations made based on it?

How to respond to case studies

Case studies in nursing and midwifery

A case study is a 'description of an actual situation, commonly involving a decision, a challenge, an opportunity, a problem, or an issue faced by a person or persons in an organization' (Leenders *et al.* 2001 cited in Popil 2011, p. 205). In education, case studies are primarily used to engage students' **content knowledge and critical thinking skills** in order for them to suggest possible solutions to the particular problem or situation.

In nursing and midwifery, case studies, also called '*clinical case scenarios*', are frequently used to assess students' ability to put theory and content knowledge into clinical application. Cases are set in clinical scenarios and require students to consider a number of variables (e.g. gender, age, ethnicity, pre-existing conditions) that play a key role in deciding an appropriate course of action and making recommendations.

Case studies thus require nursing and midwifery students to

- consider carefully the clinical context and the variables that play a key role in the case,
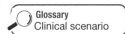
Glossary
Clinical scenario
- select relevant clinical knowledge and processes, and
- propose a care plan for the client at the centre of the case.

Preparing to respond to a case study

Before you are in a position to respond to a case study, you need to identify and examine the issues or problems presented in it. This involves three steps: understanding the context of the case (1), identifying the problems or key issues presented in the case (2), and linking theory and clinical experience to the situation described in the case (3).

1   *Understanding the context of the case*

Understanding the background of the case is essential as it will help you select the relevant clinical knowledge needed in order to suggest a care plan and make a recommendation. To gain a good understanding of the background and the issues presented in the case:

- read the case to get the gist of it first, then
- identify the key variables (e.g. gender, age, ethnicity, pre-existing conditions) affecting the patient at the centre of the case, and finally
- make notes on the background and the key variables of the case.

2 *Identifying the problems presented in the case*

Before you can suggest the best possible care plan and make recommendations, you need to identify:

- the main problems in the case,
- their relationship with the key variables you isolated in the previous step, and
- the reasons that may have caused them.

To do this, you will need to:

- list or summarize the variables, the problems, and the possible causes,
- analyse the main problems or issues,
- find evidence from the case itself that supports your analysis,
- identify the possible causes of the problems or issues, and
- outline what should be done.

> **Glossary**
> Analyse
> Identify
> Outline
> Summarize

To help you with this, you could either draw a table (Table 7.5) or a mindmap (Figure 7.4) as illustrated below:

Table 7.5 Identifying problems in case studies (table format)		
Main problems	Key variables	Possible causes
Description	Description:	Description:
	Evidence found in the case:	Action:

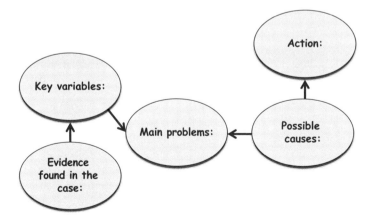

Figure 7.4 **Identifying problems in case studies (mindmap format)**

3 *Linking theory and clinical experience to the case situation*

The key purpose of this step is for you to link your knowledge of the content of your course and your previous clinical experience to the situation presented in the case. This is an opportunity to show your ability to apply theory (content knowledge, theories of nursing and midwifery, etc.) and clinical practice to a given situation. For this, you will need to:

● identify content knowledge you covered in your course that is related to the case,
● select appropriate theories that are relevant to the issues or problems presented in the case, and
● summarize how content knowledge and theories help explain the problems and the possible causes you have identified.

Note: If you decide to use references to support your choice of content knowledge and theories, remember to follow the referencing system recommended for your course (see Chapter 10).

Suggesting possible solutions and making recommendations

Once you have completed the three steps outlined above, you will be in a position to suggest solutions and make recommendations. It is worth noting that recommendations may not always be required. Similarly, it is always useful to keep in mind that there may be more than one possible solution to any given case.

To be able to identify the most appropriate solution to the problem or problems presented in the case, you will have to consider its effectiveness as well as the cost, time and resources needed to implement it. To this end, you may want to compare the solution you have identified with others that may still be relevant but less effective.

Table 7.6 Identifying the best possible solution for a case				
Solution	Effectiveness	Cost	Time	Resources
Solution 1:				
Solution 2:				
Solution 3:				

To help you with this, you can draw a table where you list the advantages and disadvantages associated with each of the solutions you have identified in relation to their effectiveness, cost, time and resources (Table 7.6).

A table like this should not only help you decide on the most appropriate solution but also provide you with information as to why other solutions are less appropriate in case you decide to provide a comparative answer.

An example

Marisa is a primigravida 43-year-old woman from Brazil, with a history of high blood pressure. As she speaks very little English she has not booked appointments before now although this is week 28 of her pregnancy.

What care should the midwife provide?

Context of the case: Patient's profile (Table 7.7)

- Primigravida, week 28 of gestation
- 43 years old
- History of blood pressure
- No previous booked appointments
- Brazilian with little English

Table 7.7 An example of main problems presented in a case study

Main problems	Key variables	Possible causes
Description: *Delayed childbearing has an increased risk of adverse pregnancy outcomes, hypertensive disorders of pregnancy may cause miscarriage as well as maternal deaths (pre-eclampsia)*	Description: *Delayed childbearing, lack of antenatal care, little English*	Description: *History of blood pressure, second half of gestation*
	Evidence: *43 years of age primigravida, no booked appointments therefore no monitoring of blood pressure*	Action: *Detecting, monitoring and controlling her blood pressure, using interpreter to make sure she understands situation and can make informed decisions in future.*

Main problems presented in the case

- Relevant content knowledge
  - Delayed childbearing
  - Hypertension in pregnancy
  - Eclampsia

- Appropriate theories and approaches
  - NICE guidelines
  - Pre-eclampsia community guideline (PRECOG)

Relevant care plan

Detecting gestational hypertension early is one of the main aims of antenatal care. As the patient did not make previous appointments, detecting, monitoring and controlling her blood pressure is imperative as the risks of her developing gestational hypertension increase in the second half of gestation. It is also important that the woman understands the situation so that she can make informed decisions. Therefore the midwife needs to:

- seek help (e.g. bilingual relative, community interpreter) to reduce the possibility of misunderstanding due to language barriers;
- identify the presence of factors (e.g. first pregnancy, age $\geq$ 40 years, body mass index $\geq$ 35, diastolic blood pressure $\geq$ 80 mm Hg) that predispose pregnant women to pre-eclampsia;
- identify the presence of signs and symptoms of the onset of pre-eclampsia such as (new) hypertension, (new) proteinuria, headache or visual disturbance, epigastric pain or vomiting, reduced foetal movements;
- monitor her blood pressure, test her urine for protein, and bring her as near to term as possible;
- (if the patient's gestational hypertension is severe), aim to control her blood pressure, refer her for early specialist input, have a thorough discussion of obstetric risk, and possibly early delivery.

How to write research proposals

Research proposals are another important type of document that you will have to write, especially when you are nearing the end of your course of study or when you start your professional career.

A research proposal is a concise and coherent summary of your proposed research. It identifies the central issues or questions that you aim to address and outlines the area of study of your research. It also locates your work within the current state of knowledge and recent debates.

A research proposal is your opportunity to:

- clarify your thinking and ideas on a research topic or area,
- create an outline for your work, and
- share your project with others.

Research proposals can serve many different functions. They can help you:

- Think through the research project you are planning and envisage possible difficulties.
- Get organized.
- Think about ways in which difficulties can be overcome.
- Anticipate possible results.
- Keep you on track once you have started your project.

Research proposals will also help you discuss your ideas with other people. They are a good starting point for discussing your work with other students, your personal tutor and your supervisor. It is important that you keep your proposal as flexible as possible so that you will be able to make room for suggestions that you think are worth accepting.

What sections should a research proposal have? It will depend on what type of research you are planning to do. An experimental project will certainly have more sections than a study based on a literature search.

Research has traditionally been divided into:

- **Field research,** also called experimental or primary research.
- **Desk research,** also called bibliographical or secondary research.

You conduct field research when you want to obtain new data to answer a specific set of questions about a topic or issue of interest. You normally use questionnaires, interviews, tasks or tests as your data-collection instruments. You then use statistical tests to measure how representative of the population at large your data are. For example, as part of your field research you may want to examine the nursing needs of minority ethnic groups in a given region of your country. You would need to design a questionnaire to use with your chosen sample of that population. You would then need to examine the results from your questionnaires using statistical tests to measure the strength of your results. In the health sciences this type of research, known as **applied research,** often seeks to improve the health care of a particular group or the treatment of a particular disease.

You conduct a piece of desk research when you need to analyse data that have already been collected by others. This involves the critical examination of sources of information such as journal articles, books, library databases, reports and government statistics. You may examine what has been published in connection with your topic so as to be able to evaluate the strength and the weaknesses of our knowledge in that area and suggest gaps in the literature that should be bridged. This is also known as **basic research** in health sciences.

Table 7.8 shows the different parts of a research proposal, together with a short description of what you should include in each section. It also indicates whether the section should be part of your proposal, depending on the type of research project you are planning.

Table 7.8   Sections of a research proposal

Section	Short description	Type	
		Field	Desk
Title page	Should contain name of university, school/ department, your name, student number, the working title of project, your supervisor's name, and the date you are handing it in.	✓	✓
Abstract	Should be a concise summary of your whole proposal. Abstracts are short and should not be confused with introductions.	✓	✓
Introduction	Should provide readers with a general description of your research, present its rationale, state the problem you want to examine, specify the steps you will take to do it (objectives) and outline what you will discuss in it (scope). Objectives should be SMART: Specific, Measurable, Attainable, Realistic and Time-oriented.	✓	✓
Research question or research hypothesis	The research question or hypothesis should define your research, provide direction to it, and act as its frame of reference.	✓	✓
Literature review	Should briefly explain what we already know about your topic, the main related concepts and theories, whether there are inconsistencies, what needs to be done (gap), and what contribution(s) you expect to make with your research.	✓	✓
Methodology	Should define the type of study you are proposing, access and ethical issues, participants and how they will be selected, data-collection instruments and methods of analysis (e.g. statistical tests). Its main aim is to provide a brief description of the methods (e.g. RCTs) you will be using in your research.	✓	Only briefly explained
Anticipated problems	Should mention problems you may anticipate (e.g. time, access to participants and resources) and consider possible strategies to solve them.	✓	✗
Timeline	Should mention how long you expect the project to last.	✓	✗

| Ethical considerations | Should include the considerations and responsibilities that you have taken in relation to the participants as well as their physical and emotional well-being. | ✓ | ✓ |
| Bibliography | Should contain the list of references you have cited in your proposal, the sources you have read but not cited, and also those you intend to read but have not yet had time to. It is important to follow the referencing system (e.g. Harvard, APA) that your department or university adheres to. | ✓ | ✓ |

Table 7.9 provides a checklist that you can use once you have finished writing your research proposal to make sure you have included all the necessary information.

Table 7.9   A checklist for the sections of a research proposal

Section	Key question	Further considerations
Title	Does the title make reference to (1) the content and (2) the context of the questions you wish to investigate?	Does it do it in a succinct – brief and clear – way?
Abstract	Does the abstract briefly summarize the what (issues or questions), the why (the importance of investigating the what), and the how (the methods you will use to investigate the what) of your proposed research? Does it also present the expected outcomes?	Is it written within the word limit (150 to 200 words)?
Introduction	Background: Does the introduction provide a background to the area of your research? Does it contextualize the research question or hypothesis? Does it provide a strong rationale for your research? Aims and objectives: Do the aims of your research explain what you want to achieve in general terms? Do the objectives support your aims in a specific way?	Does it do all this in a succinct but convincing way? Are your objectives SMART?
Research question/ hypothesis	Do the research questions or hypotheses define your research? Do they provide a direction to your research and give it a frame of reference?	Are they clearly defined, including elements such as participants, interventions, design and possible outcomes? (Also see systematic reviews)

Review of the literature	Does the review of the literature present a critical evaluation of the relevant research in the area of your study? Does it look at its strengths, weaknesses and contributions? Does it identify gaps in your area of research? Does it mention the gaps your study aims to narrow?	Does it do all this in a critical rather than summative way? (Also see argumentative writing in Chapter 6)
Methodology	Does the methodology briefly describe (1) the approach your research will follow, (2) the participants and how they will be selected, (3) the data-collection instruments that will be used, and (4) the method(s) of data analysis?	Does it do this in a descriptive rather than an argumentative manner? (Also see argumentative writing in Chapter 6)
Limitations	Does this section present a brief indication of the potential constraints (e.g. time, access to participants and resources) of your study?	Based on these limitations, is your study still feasible?
Ethical considerations	Does this section describe the considerations and responsibilities (e.g. access to full information about the study, their right to withdraw at any time and without consequences) that you have taken in relation to your participants? Does it include considerations about their physical and emotional well-being?	Do you need to provide samples of the 'Participant Information Sheet' and the 'Participant Consent Form' that you will use in an appendix?
References and Bibliography	Does this section present all the sources that you have read in preparation for the proposal? Does it follow the right referencing system? (Also see Chapter 10.)	Do you need to include relevant sources that you plan to read in the future?

How to prepare to write your undergraduate dissertation

This section of the chapter discusses how to *get prepared* to write your undergraduate dissertation. It *does not deal with dissertations* as such, for which you will have to consult your personal tutor or supervisor and other books that specifically deal with dissertation writing. Rather, this section deals with planning and organizing to write the different sections of your dissertation draft.

In your view or experience, what should be the parts of an undergraduate dissertation? Write them in the blank balloons in Figure 7.5 (add more balloons if necessary).

Compare your answers with the list shown in Table 7.8. Tick those that you included in the spidergram and cross those that you did not. You can use this as a checklist for your own work, paying closer attention to those sections for which you have selected a cross (Table 7.10).

Figure 7.5 Sections of a dissertation

Table 7.10 Sections of a dissertation		
Sections	✓	✗
Title page		
Acknowledgements		
List of contents		
Abstract		
Introduction		
Literature review		
Research methods		
Results		
Discussion		
Conclusion(s)		
References		
Appendices		

The sections in bold are common to both desk research and field research dissertations. For example, the research methods and results sections will be part of a field research dissertation, but will not normally be part of a desk research one.

The functions of each main section of a dissertation are illustrated in Table 7.11.

Table 7.11 The functions of the main sections of a dissertation	
Section	Main functions
Introduction	• Provides **background** to contextualize the problem on which your dissertation will focus • Presents the **rationale** for your research • Indicates what **gap** in our knowledge or understanding your dissertation will fill • States the **objectives** and **research questions** of your dissertation and its **scope**

Section	Main functions
Literature review	• Presents a **critical analysis** of the work already existing in your research area • Points to the **gaps** your dissertation will fill • Indicates the **contributions** your dissertation will make to the field
Research methods	• Makes reference to the **type of study** (qualitative, quantitative, mixed methods etc.) • Explains **access** and **confidentiality** issues • Indicates **arrangements of groups** (control, experimental, etc.) • Describes **instruments for data collection** used • Explains the **statistical tests** used if applicable
Results	• Discusses **findings** relating to research questions • Points to the **salient aspects** of the findings • Uses **varied methods of presentation** of findings (tables, graphs etc.)
Discussion	• Confirms or disconfirms your **hypothesis** (field research only) • Clarifies the **research questions** in the light of the results presented • Discusses the **contribution** of your research
Conclusion(s)	• Summarizes the **discussion** of results • Clarifies the **implications** of your findings • Analyses the **limitations** of your research • Suggests areas of **further research**

There are questions that can help you make sure that you have included all the relevant information in each of these sections. Such questions (Table 7.12) can serve two purposes: they can help you plan and get organized before you start writing your dissertation; and they can also be used as a checklist after you have written your first draft. Readers of your dissertation should be able to answer these questions after they have read each part of your dissertation.

Finally, when you are writing your introduction, remember that a good introduction should:

• Be **well organized** (follow the sequence given in Table 7.11).
• Include **enough detail** to whet the reader's appetite, but should not be too long.
• Specify the **problem** to be researched **clearly**.

When preparing to write the literature review, you will have to read widely. You may find it difficult to organize your notes after so much reading. Here are some organizing and writing tips for you to consider when reading for and writing your review:

• When you read, **keep an annotated bibliography**. An annotated bibliography includes a brief critical synopsis of the contents and contributions made by each of the sources you read.
• **Organize** the synopses from the annotated bibliography by theme. Relate synopses that deal with the same or a similar topic or issue together.

Table 7.12 A checklist for the main sections of a dissertation	
Section	Main questions
Introduction	• Where is this problem contextualized? And where can this problem be observed? • Why is this research important? • What is the gap in our knowledge that this research will fill? • What steps will be taken to improve the situation? • What aspects of the problem will the research discuss?
Literature review	• What is already known about the field of study? • What are the main concepts in the field? • How are these concepts related? • What theories are the most prominent in the field? • What shortcomings/inconsistencies are there in the field? • What needs to be done? • Why investigate the research problem posed in the study? • What contribution will the study make to the field?
Research methods	• What type of study is this? • Have issues of access to the data and confidentiality been addressed? • What arrangements to the groups studied or the data collected have been made? • What instruments for data collection have been used? • How have the data been analysed?
Results	• How do the findings relate to the research questions? • What are the most salient aspects of the findings?
Discussion	• Does the discussion section illuminate the research questions? • If the research is hypotheses driven, have they been confirmed or rejected? • Does the discussion section analyse the contribution that the present research makes?
Conclusion(s)	• Does the conclusion relate the findings and the discussion to the research questions? • Does it examine the implications of the findings? • Does it analyse the limitations of the study? • Does it point to areas of further research?

- **Start focused reading.** Based on the themes you have established, read sources that are directly related to these themes. Avoid reading interesting but unconnected sources.
- **Write individual sections.** Write sections – essays, if you prefer – on each of the themes that you have identified.
- **Integrate individual sections.** Analyse how the individual sections you have written relate to one another and integrate them, producing longer sections.

Revising the objectives of this chapter

Tick those objectives that you feel you have achieved and review those you have not yet managed to accomplish. Then, complete the **Achievement Chart** at the back of the book.

In this chapter, you have learnt to:

☐ write action plans

☐ write care plans

☐ prepare, write and choose an appropriate format for portfolios

☐ use a personal diary template

☐ produce reports

☐ write systematic reviews

☐ respond to case studies

☐ identify effective ways of producing research proposals

☐ plan to start writing your dissertation.

Working with Texts

In this last part of the book, you will work on variation in writing, plagiarism and referencing. You will first look at how to provide variety to your sentences and to the structure of your essays. Then you will examine plagiarism and how to avoid it. Finally, you will study the most commonly used systems of referencing in your discipline.

CHAPTER 8: VARIETY IN WRITING

Chapter 8 works at a micro level of writing. It focuses on how to add variety to sentences, use different cohesive devices to improve the flow of the texts, and achieve variety in structure within and between paragraphs. It also examines academic writing style.

CHAPTER 9: AVOIDING PLAGIARISM

In this chapter you will deal with a fundamental aspect of writing in an academic environment: plagiarism. The chapter starts by exploring what plagiarism means and why you should avoid it. The focus then is on different strategies to avoid plagiarizing other people's work.

CHAPTER 10: REFERENCING SYSTEMS

This last chapter explores the reasons for as well as the mechanics of referencing in academic writing. You will examine in-text referencing, quotations and reference lists. You will then look at how to follow referencing systems in nursing and midwifery. The chapter closes with an examination of the most commonly available bibliographical software packages, such as EndNote, RefWorks and Refbase.

Variety in Writing

At the end of this chapter, you should be able to:

- recognize different ways of adding variety to your texts
- identify different sentence openers
- use cohesive devices to support textual variety
- recognize structural elements used for adding variety between parts of a text.

Text variety

In this section of the chapter you will explore variety in texts. Variety is an important concept in writing, as it helps you produce texts that are more interesting and easier to read.

Why does variety matter? Textual variety matters for a number of reasons.

- It avoids boredom and encourages readers to keep on reading.
- It makes your ideas clearer and makes them sound more interesting.
- It shows the relationship between ideas (e.g. main and secondary).
- It avoids creating the wrong effect in the reader (e.g. a succession of very short sentences may create suspense).

Text variety can be achieved in a number of ways, and it usually results from a combination of factors. For example, it can be achieved by:

- Using **different subject forms** to avoid overusing the typical 'subject + verb' sentence opener.
- Changing the **word order** of some of the sentences to make some ideas more prominent.
- Adding **connectives** (e.g. 'and', 'however' etc.) to vary your sentence structure and length.
- Using **different sentence lengths** to write texts that are more interesting and attractive to read.

- Using related vocabulary items such as 'word families' (e.g. to ease, easy, easily) and synonymous expressions (e.g. to ease the pain, to relieve the pain) to create a lexical thread in your texts. Related words will also enhance cohesion (see Chapter 1).

Table 8.1 contains a list of these elements and how they contribute to textual variety. This list can assist you when editing your own texts. These elements will be explored in more detail in the sections of the chapter that follow.

Table 8.1 Elements in text variety	
Text element	Can help you
Subject forms	avoid repetition of sentence openers
Word order	change emphasis
Connectives	highlight the relationship between ideas
Sentence length	make your texts flow more smoothly
Related vocabulary items	add unity to your texts

ACTIVITY 8.1

Read the following two texts and then answer the questions below.

1. How do you think the texts compare?
2. Which shows more variety?
3. How do you think variety has been achieved in this text?
4. Can you underline the elements that have been used to support variety in the text?

Text 1

Nurses can work in many health-care settings. They can gain experience in all aspects of caring for clients and their families. They can build their professional career in many different ways. They may choose to become clinical specialists or consultant nurses, or they can opt for managerial positions as a head of nursing services or supervisor of other nurses. They may even prefer to pursue an academic career in education and research. These are just a few examples of the opportunities that nurses currently have to develop their professional interests.

Text 2

Nurses can work in many health-care settings, which gives them the opportunity to gain experience in all aspects of caring for clients and their families. Nurses can thus build their professional career in many different ways. For instance, they may choose to become clinical specialists or consultant nurses, or they can opt for managerial positions as a head of nursing services or supervisor of other nurses. For the more academic-oriented ones, there are also opportunities in education and research. These are just a few examples of the opportunities that nurses currently have to develop their professional interests.

Answers See suggested answers on p. 201.

Sentence variety

Varying the structure of the sentences in your texts is also important to attract your readers' attention and encourage them to keep on reading.

One common problem of unattractive texts is that they use the same sentence opener or sentence structure time and time again. For example, if a text only shows the typical sentence opener *subject + verb*, it will produce a monotonous effect and its readers will tire easily. Similarly, if the text is a group of only short and simple sentences, it will read as choppy (broken up) and will lose the interest of its readers.

Table 8.2 shows some of the most common problems connected with sentence variety and offers some alternatives to improve them. The grammar of the sentences is further explained in the section on writing style later in the chapter.

Table 8.2 Problems with sentence structure		
Problem	**Alternative 1**	**Alternative 2**
Choppy sentences	Use **coordination** (if ideas are of equal value): 'and', 'but', 'or', 'so' etc.	Use **subordination** (if one idea is dependent on the other): 'when', 'while', 'because' etc.
Same subject in various consecutive sentences	**Replace** the subject for a pronoun.	Use **relative pronouns**: 'who', 'which', 'that'.
Subject + verb pattern in various consecutive sentences	Use a **preposition** to start the sentence: **After** completing the form, the patient was directed to...	Use a **participle** to start the sentence: **Having completed** the form, the patient was directed to...

Of the problems listed in Table 8.2, lack of variety in the sentence openers is the most notorious. To avoid repeating the common sentence opener 'subject + verb', vary the form of the subject of your sentences. Here are some of the most common forms that sentences can take as subject:

- Clause: Although his case was not urgent, the patient was examined immediately.
- Adverb: Quickly and effectively, all casualties were treated by the new team of surgeons.
- Infinitive phrase: To gain a deeper understanding of the issue, the midwife gathered as much information as she possibly could.
- Participial phrase: Hoping to gain a deeper understanding of the issue, the midwife gathered as much information as she possibly could.
- Nominalization: A decision about the case was not made until the small hours of the following day.
- Cleft sentences: It was his weight loss that caught everyone's attention.

ACTIVITY 8.2

Read the following text and underline the forms of the subject that have been used to add variety to the text.

Cutting and repairing an episiotomy, and repairing vaginal/perineal lacerations were each proposed and retained as basic skills. Repairing a cervical laceration was proposed and retained as an additional skill. There is considerable Grade I evidence that avoiding episiotomy enhances both short- and long-term perineal integrity, supporting the midwifery philosophy of non-intervention. This evidence is counterbalanced by other Grade I evidence that restricting the use of episiotomy increases the risk of anterior perineal trauma.

Answers See suggested answers on p. 201.

Word order

Changing the word order of a sentence will add variety to your text too. It will also help you change the emphasis of a sentence, while calling the reader's attention to the point being made in that part of the sentence.

Consider the following two examples:

(1) She never thought she would be promoted so quickly.
(2) Never did she think she would be promoted so quickly.

In (1) the focus of information attention is placed on the second part of the sentence (quick promotion). In sentence (2), on the other hand, the emphasis falls on how unexpected the promotion was for her.

Consider these other two examples:

(3) The doctor saw her patients in Ward 2 yesterday morning.
(4) Yesterday morning the doctor saw her patients in Ward 2.

While the focus of attention in sentence (3) is on *what* happened, in sentence (4) it is on *when* it happened.

It is important to remember, though, that when you change the word order of your sentences you also change their focus of attention. Make sure that there is a good reason for doing this, and that the point you are trying to make by changing the focus of attention is clear and justifiable. Otherwise, you may create confusion in your readers.

Cohesive variety

Cohesion is what holds a text together (see Chapters 1 and 5). Cohesion is necessary not only between sentences but also between paragraphs. Cohesive variety can be achieved by using:

- Words that are related (e.g. synonymous expressions).
- Cohesive devices (e.g. finally).
- Related concepts.
- Reference to previously mentioned points (e.g. this, that).
- Substitution (e.g. substituting 'nurses' with the personal pronoun 'they').

Table 8.3 shows examples of how these elements can be used to achieve cohesiveness. Use the list to help you edit your own texts.

ACTIVITY 8.3

Read the following text and underline the elements that have been used to achieve cohesiveness.

As pressure to control hospital costs has intensified, the need to deliver the best nursing care in the most economical way has grown. Internationally research reviews show the benefits of home care. For example, dialysis patients can be reunited with their families and hospital beds used only when really necessary. In addition, by reducing hospital stays, governments undoubtedly save thousands of dollars. Nevertheless, it is not possible for professionals and policy-makers to estimate the resource implications of in-home services in Hong Kong unless systematic research is undertaken. (Luk 2002, p. 269)

Answers See suggested answers on p. 201.

Structural variety in paragraphs

The term 'structural variety' encompasses all the other aspects of variety that you have examined in the previous sections. This section shows you how they all work

Table 8.3 Cohesive elements in texts	
Cohesive element	Example
Related words	Surgical treatment for gynaecological cancer raises particular difficulties in relation to **altered fertility, changes in body image** and **sexual dysfunction**. These **problems** may, in turn, trigger a significant life crisis for the entire family. (Maughan *et al.* 2002, p. 27)
Cohesive devices	**Although** sleep disturbance is the most important and bothersome symptom experienced by these patients, there are few documented interventional studies that have addressed this problem. **Thus**, there is a need to develop effective methods to manage sleep disturbance of ESRD patients. (Tsaya & Chen 2003, p. 1)
Related concepts	All human beings need stimulation to keep their **brain functioning** in a normal way. Deprivation of stimulation leads to a **deterioration of behaviour**. There is a considerable risk that the patient in the final stage of **dementia** will get too little stimulation. (Norberg *et al.* 2003, p. 473)
This, that, these, those (to refer to previously mentioned points/ideas)	Surgical treatment for gynaecological cancer raises particular difficulties in relation to altered fertility, changes in body image and sexual dysfunction. **These** problems may, in turn, trigger a significant life crisis for the entire family. (Maughan *et al.* 2002, p. 27)
Substitution	Managers of the units were asked to inform **staff and nurses** during the ward meeting about the purpose of the investigation and asked **them** to take part in it. The questionnaires were distributed in a sealed envelope including an introductory letter and **they** were told that **their** anonymity would be preserved. (Tummers *et al.* 2002, p. 845)

together to keep the structure within and between paragraphs attractive to your readers.

In this section, you will examine how to:

- Combine long and short sentences within paragraphs.
- Provide logical connections between paragraphs.

It is important to **combine short** and **long sentences** in the same paragraph. Too many long sentences would make reading the text more demanding and may lead to confusion. Too many short sentences, on the other hand, may create a choppy effect in your text. A long sentence should be followed by a short one, especially if another long sentence will follow afterwards.

The short sentence may have several functions. It may:

- Summarize the ideas in the previous sentence.
- Provide a link between two long sentences.
- Mark a transition between the topics of two long sentences.

ACTIVITY 8.4

Read the following texts and choose one of the labels below to define the function of the sentence in italics in each of them. There is one too many labels.

| Summarize | | Link | | Mark a transition |

Text 1

Several studies suggest that brief interventions do not significantly contribute to smoking cessation during pregnancy and have concluded that interventions may benefit the foetus, but their medium-term effects on helping mothers stop smoking are inconclusive. *This seems to indicate that to be effective smoking cessation intervention should consider both the foetus and the mother.* It seems reasonable to suggest that programmes of sustained support would need to be implemented so as to help smokers not only during pregnancy but also after giving birth.

Text 2

Client-centred care, which sees the client as a holistic individual, is one of the basic principles that a nurse should learn as it underlies both the theory and the practice of nursing care. *To provide client-centred care, nurses should recognize culture-sensitive practices and their relation to social cultures.* Societal characteristics are important sources of information for nurses to be able to make informed decisions in their daily practice, as these should result from their reflection on practice and respect for ethnicity, culture and differences.

Answers See suggested answers on p. 202.

Providing **logical connections** or **relationships between paragraphs** is another way of adding textual variety, while also making transitions between the parts of your text more smooth. Logical connections can be marked by a word ('similarly'), a phrase ('on the other hand') or a whole sentence.

ACTIVITY 8.5

Read the following texts and underline the logical connections used. In some cases you don't have the preceding text, but you should still be able to identify the logical connection.

Text 1

In contrast to this prevailing view of women as objects, many international leaders and agencies have taken action to promote women as persons with full human rights, beginning with the female child. (Thompson 2002, p. 189)

Text 2

Psychiatric and Social Work pre-admission assessment have long-standing histories as requirements of UK Mental Health Acts (1983). Pre-admission nursing assessment has no such obvious legal authority; however, the practice is commonplace for most, if not all, Medium and High Security Hospitals.

Despite the widespread nature of this practice, pre-admission nursing assessments have received little descriptive or research attention in forensic mental health. (Watt *et al.* 2003, p. 645)

Text 3

The women in the midwifery group were seen by an obstetrician during their initial visit to the midwives' clinic and at 36 weeks' gestation to confirm their low-risk status.

Apart from the two mandatory obstetrician visits, the midwives made autonomous decisions on the care they provided. They made referrals to, or consulted with, obstetricians and other health team members when the need arose. (Harvey *et al.* 2002, p. 262)

Answers See suggested answers on p. 202.

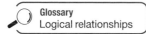

Glossary
Logical relationships

You should provide logical connections between paragraphs when you want to:

- Show comparison or contrast between the two parts of your text (e.g. using 'however' for contrast and 'similarly' for comparison).
- Enumerate reasons or examples.
- Produce a counter-argument (e.g. using a concession: *although these cases have clearly been reviewed, there are still some inconclusive results that require further examination*).

Writing style

All of the different elements we discussed in the previous sections constitute what we call 'writing style'. They can be grouped into three basic principles that should guide your academic writing:

- simplicity;
- brevity;
- logic.

Each of these principles can be achieved in a number of ways. *Simplicity*, for example, has to do with sentence length and choice of words. *Logic* is the result of careful planning, using the right connectives and following grammatical principles such as agreement. We will now analyse each of these principles in more detail.

Simplicity

One way of keeping your writing simple is by monitoring the length of your sentences. This, of course, doesn't mean that all your sentences should be short and simple. As discussed above, a succession of short sentences will give your text a choppy style or create an effect of suspense that you surely want to avoid in your academic essays. On the other hand, too many complex sentences together will tire your reader. What you should try to do is to combine short and long sentences, which will add variety to your text, making it easy and pleasant to read. Compare the three examples in Figure 8.1.

Example 1: A succession of short sentences

Many studies have produced inconclusive evidence in relation to smoking cessation during pregnancy (e.g. Kelley *et al.* 2001; Melvin *et al.* 2000; Melvin & Gaffney 2004). Several of these studies suggest that brief interventions do not contribute to smoking cessation during pregnancy (Fiore *et al.* 2000; Lumley *et al.* 2004). Lawrence *et al.* (2005) have forcefully concluded that some programmes may benefit the foetus but not the mother. This seems to indicate that smoking cessation in pregnancy is unsuccessful because support to the woman is only occasional and lacks structure. Programmes of sustained support would need to be implemented during pregnancy and after birth. These programmes should then be structured in a way that offers both in-pregnancy and post-partum support.

Example 2: A succession of long and complex sentences

Although many studies have produced inconclusive evidence in relation to smoking cessation during pregnancy (e.g. Kelley *et al.* 2001; Melvin *et al.* 2000;

Melvin & Gaffney 2004), several seem to suggest that brief interventions do not contribute to smoking cessation during pregnancy (Fiore *et al.* 2000; Lumley *et al.* 2004). Lawrence *et al.* (2005) have forcefully concluded that some programmes may benefit the foetus but not the mother, which seems to indicate that smoking cessation in pregnancy is unsuccessful because support to the woman is only occasional and lacks structure and thus programmes of sustained support would need to be implemented during pregnancy and after birth, and should be structured in a way that offers both in-pregnancy and post-partum support.

Example 3: A combination of short and long sentences

Many studies have produced inconclusive evidence in relation to smoking cessation during pregnancy (e.g. Kelley *et al.* 2001; Melvin *et al.* 2000; Melvin & Gaffney 2004). Several of these studies suggest that brief interventions do not contribute to smoking cessation during pregnancy (Fiore *et al.* 2000; Lumley *et al.* 2004). Lawrence *et al.* (2005) have forcefully concluded that some programmes may benefit the foetus but not the mother, which seems to indicate that smoking cessation in pregnancy is unsuccessful because support to the woman is only occasional and lacks structure. Thus, programmes of sustained support would need to be implemented during pregnancy as well as after birth. These programmes should then be structured in a way that offers both in-pregnancy and post-partum support.

Figure 8.1 **Sentence length**

Choice of words will also contribute to keeping your style simple. This does not mean that you should avoid using 'technical vocabulary' that is part of the lexicon of your discipline. Technical words may appear complex at first, but these are the words that your readers expect to find in your writing. What is more, technical words are very difficult to replace, as they have become part of the technical vocabulary used to write about your discipline. As opposed to general and vague words (e.g. thing, it, nice), accurate and specific words will always contribute positively to your writing style.

If this is the first time that you are writing an assignment on a topic with which you are not very familiar, it is always a good idea to start collecting words that recur in your reading sources. These words make up the core technical vocabulary that you will need to use for your writing to be accurate and precise.

Look at the two examples in Figure 8.2. The technical or precise words in the first text have been underlined and replaced with less accurate ones in text 2.

Example 1: Accurate and precise

Post-partum haemorrhage (PPH) has been identified as one of the main complications of the third stage which accounts for the highest maternal mortality and morbidity. As demonstrated in this care, there is compelling evidence that lends support to the benefits of active management of the third stage.

Example 2: General and vague

Blood loss after birth has been identified as one the main things that may happen in the third stage which accounts for the highest level of death and disease. As demonstrated in this care, there are a lot of examples that show the benefits of active participation of the midwife in the third stage.

Figure 8.2 **Accuracy and precision**

Brevity

This is also connected to simplicity and to the principle of economy, which will improve the readability of your writing. Brevity also has to do with the selection and organizational principles that you studied in Chapter 1. The more focused – that is, free from loosely connected ideas and words – your writing becomes, the more effective the impact it will create on your readers. Keep it simple and avoid superfluous elements that will add words but no meaning to your sentences.

Logic

Logic also depends on selection and organization. A logical writing style is one in which the ideas – and the sentences used to express those ideas – flow smoothly. As we discussed above, if the first idea in your paragraph is complex and has been presented in a complex sentence, you will need to flesh out its meaning in two or probably three short and simple sentences. Coupled with this combination, you will need connectives to reinforce the logical organization of your writing.

   Agreement between subject and verb will also make your writing more logical and cohesive. If the subject and the verb of a sentence do not agree, this will create confusion in the reader's mind. Consider the following example:

- **Poor style:** Doctor Jones, after seeing all his patients, go home. (Who goes home? The doctor or his patients?)
- **Improved:** Doctor Jones, after seeing all his patients, goes home.

Similarly, if the subject of a sentence is later referred to by a pronoun that does not agree with it, it will also create confusion, making your writing less logical. Consider another example:

- **Poor style**: Nurses will always make sure that his clients receive the most beneficial care. (What does 'his' refer to?)
- **Improved**: Nurses will always make sure that their clients receive the most beneficial care.

Finally, the way in which you structure your sentences will also contribute positively to your style. When possible, it may also be a good idea to avoid:

- Starting sentences with a connective, especially with 'and', 'but' or 'because'.
- Finishing sentences with prepositions.
- Splitting infinitives (see Figure 8.3).

Example 1: Starting sentences with a connective

Poor style: There are a few intervention programmes to treat clients with a dual diagnosis. **But** they are relatively new and have not been objectively evaluated for their effectiveness. **And** increasing attention to these issues is being paid in some countries and, as a result, several integrated-approach treatment programmes have been established.

Improved: There are a few intervention programmes to treat clients with a dual diagnosis. However, they are relatively new and have not been objectively evaluated for their effectiveness. In some countries increasing attention to these issues is being paid and, as a result, several integrated-approach treatment programmes have been established.

Example 2: Finishing sentences with prepositions

Poor style: These are some of the issues they have been writing **about**.

Improved: These are some of the issues **about which** they have been writing.

Example 3: Splitting infinitives

Poor style: The nurse wanted **to systematically examine** the care that patients received in that ward.

Improved: The nurse wanted **to examine systematically** the care that patients received in that ward.

Figure 8.3 **Things to avoid when structuring sentences**

The examples in Table 8.4 show how these problems can easily be avoided to enhance your writing style.

Table 8.4 Enhancing your writing style		
Sentence grammar	Explanation	Example
Coordination	Coordination refers to the process of putting two or more ideas of **equal value** together. They could be written as separate sentences and would still make sense. The main coordinators are 'and', 'but', 'so' and 'or'.	Patients were administered their medication regularly **and** were given the list of activities they had to carry out on a daily basis.
Subordination	Subordination refers to putting together two or more unequal ideas (**one is dependent – D – on the other**). If written separately, one would not make complete sense. Subordinators include 'although', 'unless', 'if' and 'because'.	**Because** she was so tired at the end of the shift (D), she decided to go straight to bed.
Clause	A group of words, one of which is a finite (conjugated) verb.	**At the end of the shift she was so tired that she decided to go straight to bed.**
Phrase	A group of words without a finite verb.	**A group of student midwives.**
Infinitive phrase	A phrase whose main word is an infinitive verb.	**To support his patient emotionally** was all that the GP worried about at that moment.
Participial phrase	A phrase whose main word is an -ed or -ing word, or a word that has the same form as the past participle of irregular verbs (e.g. hidden).	**Hidden under a pile of other forms**, his admission form laid on the desk.

Grammar and English use

This last section of the chapter deals with some of the main grammar and language-use problems that many students experience when writing academically – see Table 8.5. If you need more detail on any of these topics, see the Glossary of Key Terms and the list of Further Readings and Resources at the end of the book.

Table 8.5 Writing academically		
Sentence grammar	Explanation	Example
Prepositional phrase	A phrase whose main word is a preposition.	**On performing a pelvic examination**, she discovered that the pregnancy was ectopic.
Nominalization	The process by which a verb or adjective is turned into a noun, resulting in an impersonal structure.	There is **a demand** for further discussions about pregnancy termination.
Cleft sentences	Sentences that have two parts (and two finite verbs). They are useful to call the reader's attention to the first part of the sentence.	**What we now need** are actions more than words.
Fragment	A phrase or incomplete sentence that is punctuated as a complete sentence would be.	**As she was experiencing acute pain and heavy bleeding.**

Revising the objectives of this chapter

Tick those objectives that you feel you have achieved and review those you have not yet managed to accomplish. Then, complete the **Achievement Chart** at the back of the book.

In this chapter, you have learnt to:

☐ recognize different ways of adding variety to your texts

☐ identify different sentence openers

☐ use cohesive devices to support textual variety

☐ recognize structural elements used for adding variety between parts of a text.

Avoiding Plagiarism

At the end of this chapter, you should be able to:

- recognize what constitutes plagiarism and what does not
- deal with definitions and concepts already well established in your field
- paraphrase other people's ideas and words without plagiarizing.

Exploring plagiarism

What do you already know about plagiarism? Complete Figure 9.1 with some words or phrases you associate with it.

Figure 9.1 **What is plagiarism (your definitions)?**

Now read the definitions of plagiarism in Figure 9.2. Look especially at the words in bold. Did you write any of these words in your diagram?

As the definition says, plagiarism comprises two acts: stealing someone else's work and lying about it afterwards. You can avoid plagiarism by being academically honest. Don't steal, and don't lie.

According to the Merriam-Webster Online Dictionary, to 'plagiarize' means:
1) to steal and pass off (the ideas or words of another) as one's own
2) to use (another's production) without crediting the source
3) to commit literary theft
4) to present as new and original an idea or product derived from an existing source.
In other words, plagiarism is an act of fraud. It involves both stealing someone else's work and lying about it afterwards.

Figure 9.2 What is plagiarism (others' definitions)?
Source: What is Plagiarism (n.d.), www.plagiarism.org.

Plagiarism may take many different forms and sometimes students plagiarize without knowing. You could be severely penalized for plagiarism if you do any of the following. Look at the list in Table 9.1 and put a tick against those that you can identify as plagiarism and a cross against those that you didn't know about.

Some of these acts can be more easily identified as plagiarism than others. For instance, you may think that *paying somebody to write for you* (number 3) is dishonest but not plagiarism. However, if you do this you are buying somebody else's ideas and words and then pretending they are your own. This *is* plagiarism.

Changing only a few words from the original (number 6) is another form of plagiarism that you may not be so sure about. But if you change just a few words without acknowledging the original source, the words are yours but the ideas are certainly not. It's similar to number 8, *Changing the words in the original but keeping the essential ideas without citing.*

Table 9.1 Acts of plagiarism		
Acts	Knew (✓)	Didn't know (✗)
1. Handing in somebody else's work as your own.		
2. Buying or borrowing somebody else's work.		
3. Paying somebody to write for you.		
4. Copying without citing.		
5. Failing to use quotation marks.		
6. Changing only a few words from the original.		
7. Building on somebody else's ideas without giving credit.		
8. Changing the words in the original but keeping the essential ideas without citing.		
9. Paraphrasing without citing.		

Why do students plagiarize? Some believe that they are incapable of producing work worth reading or worth a good mark. They cannot see themselves as prepared to meet their tutors' expectations, so they plagiarize in the hope that they will get a pass mark. Others find it contradictory that, while they have to produce work with a certain degree of originality, they still have to reference previous work in the field (see Chapter 10).

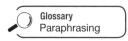
Glossary
Paraphrasing

The rest of this chapter deals with strategies for avoiding plagiarism. More specifically, you will look at strategies for dealing with established definitions and concepts, and paraphrasing.

ACTIVITY 9.1

You will read one original text and three other texts that have incorporated the original one. Determine which of the three texts plagiarizes and which does not. Be prepared to back up your choices.

Original text

Despite the difficulties faced by male partners of seriously ill women, their needs may not be recognised. Rees *et al.* (1998) assessed the information needs of nine male partners of women with breast cancer, using focus group methodology. They found that partners varied considerably in their information needs, but that health professionals generally ignored their information needs. Although this study provides a valuable insight into the information needs of partners and health professional responses, the results cannot necessarily be generalised because of the small size of the sample (Maughan *et al.* 2002, p. 28).

Text 1

Several studies have suggested that the difficulties faced by male partners of seriously ill women may not be recognized (Rees *et al.* 1998; Maughan *et al.* 2002).

Text 2

In a small study of the information needs of male partners of seriously ill women, Rees *et al.* (1998, cited in Maughan *et al.* 2002, p. 28) found that health professionals tended to pay little attention to these men's needs.

Text 3

Maughan *et al.* (2002) state that although male partners of seriously ill women face difficulties, their needs may not be acknowledged.

Answers See suggested answers on p. 203.

Dealing with definitions and concepts

One common misconception about referencing and paraphrasing is thinking that you cannot 'reproduce' what others have already said because if you do, your work will lack 'originality'. However, sometimes you are better off reproducing what others before you have said. You just have to make sure that you do it properly.

One such case is when dealing with established concepts in the field that you are researching. If, for example, you are working with the concept of 'reflection' in nursing, people reading your essay would probably expect you to refer to Gibbs' well-established model. Similarly, if your essay was on 'problem-based nursing', you would need to make reference to problem-based learning components and problem-solving processes. These cases allow you to show or display your knowledge of the field and its main contributors (also see Chapter 10).

Another reason for reproducing established ideas and concepts is connected with 'specificity'. Some definitions are highly technical and specific and a paraphrase may not cover all the specific aspects or may fail to convey the same meanings. Think, for example, how difficult it would be to provide synonymous words or phrases for 'fertilisation', 'fertility' or 'fertilised' in the following definition:

> In Vitro Fertilisation (IVF) is one of several assisted conception techniques available to help people with fertility problems to have a baby. It involves an egg being surgically removed from the ovary and fertilised outside the body. (*Health Encyclopaedia*, NHS Direct Online)

Providing a new working definition of IVF may prove not only difficult but also unnecessary. Definitions that have been accepted by the professional community have the purpose of making it possible for community members to communicate in an economical and effortless way.

It is important to remember that, to avoid plagiarism, you will need to quote the source from which you took the given definition, as shown above in relation to IVF. For a discussion and explanation of how to quote sources correctly, see Chapter 10.

Paraphrasing

Paraphrasing is an effective way of using your own words to report what others have said and offers the possibility of adding variety to your text.

A text that is heavily quoting from other sources not only lacks originality but is also uninviting to read. A healthy combination of quotations, in-text referencing (see Chapter 10) and paraphrasing will make a text more attractive to the reader.

However, you must keep in mind that changing only a few words from the original does not represent paraphrasing and may be considered plagiarism (see the first section of this chapter). When you paraphrase you change the words and sometimes the structure of the original (the form of the quote) but keep the original meanings intact. Paraphrasing thus entails summarizing and referencing. The paraphrase should be shorter and normally more focused than the original text. For this, it is always a good idea to try to concentrate on one central idea to paraphrase. The resulting paraphrase should also acknowledge the source where the original text was found.

Here are some ideas for practising paraphrasing original texts:

- Read the original text until you are sure that you understand it fully.
- Count the number of words in the original or use the word count function if you are reading an online document.
- Underline or highlight main and secondary ideas.
- Focus on the main ideas.
- Write the main ideas in your own words.
- Compare your paraphrase with the original.
- If you have used more than 10% of the words in the original, it is *not* a paraphrase and you must go back to reading the original again.

ACTIVITY 9.2

Read the following definition of Chlamydia and decide if the writers of Texts 1 and 2 have made the right choice when paraphrasing the definition in their texts. What would you have done?

Definition

Chlamydia is a common sexually transmitted disease (STD) caused by the bacterium, Chlamydia trachomatis, which can damage a woman's reproductive organs (*Health Encyclopaedia*, NHS Direct Online).

Text 1

Chlamydia, an infection that is sexually transmitted, is caused by the bacterium Chlamydia trachomatis.

Text 2

An STD caused by a bacterium, Chlamydia can damage a woman's reproductive organs.

Answers See suggested answers on p. 203.

Let us look at an example (Table 9.2). In this example you will first read the original text, then a paraphrase of the original and finally a plagiarized version.

Table 9.2 Paraphrasing and plagiarizing I	
Original	Reported
Midwifery care is *personalized* care. Within the parameter of safety the midwife upholds, she recognizes wellness as an amorphous state with periodic deviations from normal; her task is to decipher the unique and fluid patterns of each mother's well-being. The more thorough and continuous her care, the more likely she will be to detect a complication at its inception. And the better she and the mother communicate, the more readily will they develop and implement a solution. (Davis 2004, p. 5) [77 words]	PARAPHRASED ✓ One essential responsibility of the midwife is to safely discover patterns of well-being that are individual to each of her clients. This, supported by ongoing care and good communication, will allow her to discover complications early and solve them promptly. (Davis 2004, p. 5) [40 words] PLAGIARIZED ✗ Midwives offer *personalized* care. Midwives' main task is to be able to recognize the patterns of well-being of their clients. To detect complications as soon as they start and to implement solutions readily, midwives should provide continuous care and establish a relationship based on good communication with each of their clients. [51 words]

Notice that the plagiarized version not only uses many words that are the same as in the original (underlined in the plagiarized version), but also **fails to acknowledge the original source**. It shows the two features of plagiarism discussed earlier in the chapter: it *steals* and it *lies*.

Let us examine another example (Table 9.3). In this example, you will read the original text and two other versions. The lifted (plagiarized) text in the new versions has been underlined. Comments on the two new versions are given below the texts.

Table 9.3 Paraphrasing and plagiarizing II	
Version 1	Version 2
The midwives in the Swedish study approached their professional task as providers of care for the individual woman only. This can be analysed as a deviation from the idea that midwives should care for the family as a whole and encourage families to participate in the process of delivery. Besides, the midwives used the pronoun 'we' as representing the Swedish health-care system as opposed to the word 'them' when they spoke about immigrants from traditionally female genital mutilation (FGM) practising cultures.	In their study of a group of Swedish midwives, Widmark *et al.* (2002, p. 122) found that the midwives they observed showed a different approach to their professional tasks. This group of midwives preferred a more woman-only oriented approach to providing care, which differed from the traditional family-oriented approach. They also noted that the midwives polarized the descriptions of their relationship with their clients by referring to themselves as representatives of the Swedish health-care system with the pronoun 'we', and their FGM practising clients with the pronoun 'them'.

Comments	**Comments**
This is a clear example of a plagiarized text. Except for the first sentence, which has been minimally changed, the text consists of almost entirely lifted text (underlined text). The alterations here can be said to be 'cosmetic changes' and there are no bibliographical references to the original text.	This is an example of a good paraphrase. It shows a change not only in the words but also the structures used in the original text. Nevertheless, it has still managed to keep the same meanings as in the original.

Original text

The midwives in this context appeared to define themselves as advocates for the individual woman, and not as advocates or caregivers for the family as a whole. This can be interpreted as a deviation from an ideology of caring for the family as a whole, implemented in routines of educational programmes for couples antenatally and encouragement of family participation during delivery for Swedish couples. In addition, the midwives often used the word 'we' and spoke of themselves as representatives of the Swedish health care system and/or society, versus the word 'them' used when speaking about immigrants from traditionally FGM practising cultures, thus illustrating an impression of polarisation (Widmark *et al.* 2002, p. 122).

You can signpost your paraphrase by using:

- A phrase that refers to the original source (see the first sentence of version 2 in Table 9.3).
- An appropriate verb or verb phrase (e.g. *suggest, criticize, contradict* etc.; see later in this chapter).

ACTIVITY 9.3

Read the original text and the lifted version. What changes would you make to change the lifted version into a paraphrase?

Original text

The introduction of a funded midwifery pilot programme in a community where midwifery was not otherwise available provided a unique opportunity to compare the quality of midwifery care with existing maternity services for women at low obstetric risk. The safety of midwifery practice was a major concern in a region that had not experienced midwifery services. (Harvey *et al.* 2002, p. 261)

Lifted version

A funded pilot programme in midwifery support in a community where this support was not available provided the authors an excellent opportunity to compare this service with that of existing maternity services for women at low obstetric risk. One of the major concerns in the region, probably as a result of not having this kind of care before, related to safety.

Answers *See suggested answers on p. 203.*

Grammar and English use

In Tables 9.4, 9.5 and 9.6, you will find more about paraphrasing. Table 9.4 deals with structural paraphrase and Table 9.5 with lexical paraphrase. Table 9.6 explains signposting a paraphrase. If you need more detail on any of these topics, see the Glossary of Key Terms and the list of Further Readings and Resources at the end of the book.

Structural paraphrase

It is sometimes difficult to change the structure of the original text without altering its meaning. However, a paraphrase does not follow the original structure, so you must learn ways of changing the structure while keeping the original ideas and concepts. The examples in Table 9.4 should give you an idea of how structural paraphrase works.

Table 9.4 Structural paraphrase		
Change	Details	Example
The order of the parts of the sentence	Adverbials can be moved to front position with only a little change in meaning.	*Original*: They required a rest after their 48-hour shift. *Paraphrase*: After working for two days, they needed to rest.
The voice of the original text	From active to passive or from passive to active.	*O*: They provide patient care on an ongoing basis. *P*: Continuous care is provided to patients.
The length of the sentences (1)	Join ideas together to make the new sentence shorter and more concise.	*O*: Not only will they work long hours, but they will also earn less. *P*: They will be asked to work longer, but will get less money.
The length of the sentences (2)	Alternatively, you may want to expand phrases for clarity.	*O*: Not having worked in the private sector before, the midwife was unsure of some of the regulations.

Change	Details	Example
		P: The midwife had not worked in the private sector before so she was unclear about some regulations.
The length of the sentences (3)	Abridge a clause to a phrase (but see dangling modifiers in Chapter 1).	O: When they entered the operating theatre, the patient was ready for the operation. P: On entering the operating theatre, they found their patient ready for the operation.
Change connectives	Use similar connectives from the same class (and, so, but, or).	O: The nurse had finished his shift but stayed on to help. P: Although he had finished his shift, the nurse stayed on and helped.

ACTIVITY 9.4

Read the following original and reported texts and evaluate whether the reported texts are examples of **paraphrasing** or **plagiarizing**.

 Original

Original	Reported	Evaluation
Coping is a dynamic process that functions to promote survival and adaptation in response to stimuli appraised as threatening. Coping strategies are learned patterns of behavior influenced by personality traits, historical patterns of relationship, and situational stressors (Folkman & Greer 2000). Successful coping and adaptation can be promoted by stimulating belief in the personal power to control life circumstances, creating achievable goals, and generating a positive mood (Folkman & Greer 2000). (Kravits *et al.* 2010, p. 131)	Threatening stimuli may trigger coping mechanisms as a response to adapt and survive (Kravits *et al.* 2010). As Folkman and Greer (2000, cited in Kravits *et al.* 2010) have indicated, these mechanisms are learnt behaviours that depend on personality traits, previous relationships and situational stressors. Folkman and Greer (2000) have also suggested that personal control over life circumstances, attainable goals and positive mood can lead to successful coping with threatening stimuli.	

Answers See suggested answers on p. 204.

B Original	Reported	Evaluation
In the current health care environment, midwives need to know the effectiveness of interventions so informed decisions can be made about the use and distribution of limited resources. Evidence based practice (EBP) involves integrating current best research evidence with clinical expertise and patient values to make decisions about the care of patients (Sackett *et al.* 2000). In this way, research based evidence is an important vehicle to improve practice and outcomes (Ingersoll 2000). (Creedy *et al.* 2002, p. 3)	In the present environment of health care, most midwives have to know interventions that are effective so that they can make effective decisions. Evidence-based practice gives an example. It entails bringing together research evidence, clinical expertise and what patients value to provide the best care for them. As Ingersoll (2000) puts it, 'research based evidence is an important vehicle to improve practice and outcomes'.	

Answers *See suggested answers on p. 204.*

ACTIVITY 9.5

A summary of dos and don'ts about paraphrasing text

Put a tick, a cross or a question mark next to each of the following statements to indicate whether it is correct (✓), incorrect (✗) or you're not sure (?)

To paraphrase you have to	✓	✗	?
1. Read the original and change a few words.			
2. Read the original, underline the main ideas and rewrite them in your own words.			
3. Summarize the main ideas in your own words.			
4. Summarize the original text, mostly using the same words.			
5. Change some of the ideas in the original text, but use your own words.			
6. Keep the ideas in the original text and express them in your own words.			

Answers *See suggested answers on p. 204.*

Now, correct those that you have marked as incorrect.

To paraphrase you have to _____

_____

_____

_____

_____

_____

Answers See suggested answers on p. 205.

Lexical paraphrase

It may also be difficult to change the words of the original text without altering its meaning. However, as with the structure of a text, you must try to maintain the original meanings. Also remember to leave shared language (language that is not specific to the original text, e.g. 'nurses' or 'midwives') unchanged. Be aware that it may not be possible to change very specific vocabulary items.

Table 9.5 Lexical paraphrase		
Change	Details	Example
Individual words using synonymous expressions	Use a thesaurus and a dictionary.	*Original*: Stopping the habit is essential to the pregnant smoker. *Paraphrase*: It is crucial for the pregnant woman to stop smoking.
Word forms	Nouns to verbs, verbs to nouns, adjectives to adverbs.	*O*: To discover a complication at its inception is fundamental in the health sciences. *P*: The early discovery of complications is an essential aspect of health sciences.

Signposting a paraphrase

Introduce your paraphrase by using a phrase that links your text to the original or an appropriate verb. Remember to use verbs that show your analytical ability. Table 9.6 shows you some examples.

Table 9.6 Signposting a paraphrase	
Signposting phrase/verb	Example
In (their/his/her) (study/ research/work/essay)	**In her 1994 study**, Markus showed that ...
According to ...	**According to Davis's study** (2004), effective communication between the midwife and her client ...
In line with	**In line with** the framework for analysis described by Peterson (2003, p. 34) as ...
Argue	Peterson (2003, p. 34) **argues** that a convincing way of ...
Claim	Widmark *et al.* (2002) **claim** that their group of midwives polarized ...
Observe	Davis (2004) **observes** that early detection of complications will result in ...
Prove	In her study, Campbell (2004) **proved** that most of the methods previously used to determine the degree of ...
Reject	Lawrence *et al.* (2005, p. 115) seem to **reject** the idea that as administered at present smoking-cessation programmes can have any long-term effect on the pregnant smoker.
Suggest	Aston *et al.* (2006) **suggest** that regular interdisciplinary surgical morning meetings (SMM) can contribute to interdisciplinary communication significantly.

Revising the objectives of this chapter

Tick those objectives that you feel you have achieved and review those you have not yet managed to accomplish. Then, complete the **Achievement Chart** at the back of the book.

In this chapter, you have learnt to:

☐ recognize what constitutes plagiarism and what does not

☐ deal with definitions and concepts already well established in your field

☐ paraphrase other people's ideas and words without plagiarizing.

Referencing Systems

At the end of this chapter, you should be able to:

- recognize the basic principles of referencing
- identify the main referencing conventions of the Harvard, the APA and the Vancouver systems
- engage with sources
- recognize the basic uses of bibliographical software programs.

The basics of referencing

Referencing is an essential part of academic writing. Many of your ideas and arguments will need to be supported by the ideas or arguments presented by others before you. References provide a link between your work and the work that others have previously done. They show your readers that your ideas are well founded. Used in this way, references add credibility to your work.

References also demonstrate how your work contributes to developing ideas in your specific field. Many of your ideas or arguments will be elaborations on work done by others. Referencing helps you show your readers how you have built your own arguments, supporting certain views and ideas and challenging others.

You also need to reference your work to:

- Acknowledge the work of others.
- Show your reader that you have read up in your field (knowledge display).
- Avoid plagiarizing the work of others.

Use the following labels to identify the purpose(s) of referencing in the texts below. One text may accommodate more than one label.

| 1. Anchoring the text in the field | | 2. Supporting ideas |

| 3. Adding credibility | | 4. Building an argument |

Text A

Reflection has been identified as an extremely useful skill for nurses (Durgahee 1996; Johns 1996; Mountford & Rogers 1996). Schon (1991), for example, defines reflection as learning from events experienced during a practical professional experience.

Text B

Reflection is considered an appropriate vehicle for the analysis of professional practice. This analysis helps professionals understand the nature of their work and adopt a critical approach to their professional activity (Gould & Masters 2004).

Text C

Many arguments have been advanced in favour of the benefits of returning a patient with a stroke to the open-plan unit (Brown 1999; Willis 2002; Thompson 2004). These include the positive support reported by the patients and the quality of the follow-up care. However, the advantages of allowing patients with a stroke to stay in the same room have not been fully examined (Allen 2001).

Answers See suggested answers on p. 205.

Some students find the practice of referencing somehow contradictory. Whereas you have to show a certain degree of originality, you are also supposed to anchor your work in the existing literature. Similarly, you are expected to make a significant contribution of your own but you still have to give credit to the work of others.

Let us try to spell out these apparent contradictions.

Contradiction 1: Show you have done your research, but write something new and original

One of the reasons you need to reference your academic work is to show that you have 'done your homework'; that is, you have read the literature connected to the topic you are researching. However, merely putting together pieces of what others have said is not enough. You also need to provide something new. This 'something new' need not be absolutely original; after all, 'there is nothing new under the sun'. But you should always try to offer a new approach or a different way of looking at things. This contradiction can be solved by adopting the *scaffolding technique*, by which you construct new arguments on the basis of previous, more established ones. In the example in Table 10.1 the writer has used the scaffolding technique. S/he has put forward a new argument by referring to what was previously established in relation to reflection.

Table 10.1 Scaffolding	
Established arguments	Reflection has been the focus of several studies that have contributed to making it an integral part of the professional nursing practice. In his seminal work, Gibbs (1988) established not only the nature but also the importance of reflection for professional advancement. In a similar manner, Durgahee (1998), elaborating on Gibbs' contribution, examined the application of reflection to nursing.
New development	More recently, Johns (2004) has suggested that the main characteristics of reflection include reflexivity, understanding and empowerment and that these aspects have to be taught to professionals in training. Johns' arguments point to the need for teaching student nurses to reflect and for incorporating reflection activity into the learning process. Introducing students to reflection at an early stage of their training may contribute to a higher degree of reflexivity in professional practice. This essay will present an argument for the early ...

Contradiction 2: Appeal to experts and authorities, but improve on or disagree with them

Another reason you need to reference your work is to revisit critically what has been done in the field so as to help it develop. If you merely cite or summarize what has already been said, you are only repeating what is known or given. You also need to improve on what has already been established and, if necessary, be prepared to disagree with it in a critical but constructive manner. This contradiction can be resolved by using the *critical stance technique*, by means of which you provide a critique of what has been done, highlighting its strengths and pointing to ways in which its weaknesses can be improved. This is illustrated in Table 10.2.

Table 10.2 Critical stance	
Previous research	Previous studies on geropsychiatric units have focused on the complexity of the care needs of older patients (Brown 2001), the social and financial difficulties they experience (Allen 2000) and the specific admission and discharging processes they require (Alexander 1999).
New contribution	Despite these contributions, research on the needs of the practitioners in this specialized field of nursing care has been scant (Smith *et al.* 2005). This essay will examine these needs, provide a taxonomy and finally...

Contradiction 3: Improve your writing by mimicking what you hear and read, but use your own words, your own voice

There are two sides to this contradiction: mimicking and breaking new ground. When you have to produce a piece of writing you have never produced before, it is always a good idea to look at how more seasoned writers do it. You can look at the way in which they organize information, what they include in each part of their piece of writing, the language and the style they use. This is mimicking. The other side of this contradiction refers to what we call breaking new ground. When you write, you first try to reach common ground with your readers by using what is known to them; that is, by using the information and the language that you share with your readers. However, you definitely have to resort to your own voice when breaking new ground. This contradiction can be resolved by using the *old and new ground technique*. For example, you use impersonal structures (e.g. in the passive voice) for what is shared and your own voice (e.g. in the active voice) for what is new. Table 10.3 illustrates this technique.

Table 10.3　Old and new ground	
Common ground, impersonal structures	It has been argued that for smoking cessation during pregnancy to be successful, support to the pregnant smoker has to be structured and sustained (Lumley *et al.* 2004; Melvin & Gaffney 2004). Similarly, it has been forcefully argued that programmes of support should consider in-pregnancy as well as post-partum support
New ground, writer's voice	(Lawrence *et al.* 2005). This essay argues that unless support for pregnant smokers incorporates strategies by which they learn about the risks of maternal smoking to the foetus and the infant and develop cognitive and behavioural strategies for stopping, it will continue making only a marginal impact on smoking cessation during pregnancy.

Contradiction 4: Give credit where credit is due, but make your own significant contribution

This final contradiction summarizes the preceding ones. It refers to the fact that you must reference when you are borrowing other people's ideas and/or words, but you can't merely produce a summary of what has been previously done or said. You also need to help advance the field by making a new and significant contribution or by presenting a new approach to an already established topic.

Read the following texts and decide what technique has been used to develop them.

Text 1

Vaginal examination on admission and during labour is probably one of the most common procedures performed by midwives. These examinations have been studied in terms of when they should be performed and how frequently (Gibb 1991; Lefeber & Voorhoeve 1998). There has been, however, a noticeable paucity of studies examining women's feelings and experiences of vaginal examinations (Lai & Levy 2002). This critique analyses...

Text 2

Much has been written about the psychological and emotional effects of gynaecological cancer on women. Effects on altered fertility and sexual dysfunction (Anderson *et al.* 1992; Cull *et al.* 1993) have long been recognized in the literature. The psychological and emotional effects on the male partners of women with gynaecological cancer have, however, received very little attention (Maughan *et al.* 2002). This essay explores the emotional effects on male partners and...

Answers See suggested answers on p. 205.

Referencing systems

Now that we have discussed the reasons for referencing, let us have a look at its mechanics. There are two types of referencing system used:

- author–date systems (e.g. Harvard system and APA);
- numerical systems (e.g. Chicago and Vancouver systems).

An example following an author–date system would look like Table 10.4.

Table 10.4 Author–date system	
Text	Reflection has proved essential for the professional development of nurses (Gibbs 1988).
List of references	Gibbs, G. (1988) *Learning by doing. A guide to teaching and learning methods.* Further Education Unit. Oxford: Oxford Polytechnic.

The same example but following a numerical system would look like Table 10.5.

Table 10.5 Numerical system	
Text	Reflection has proved essential for the professional development of nurses. [1]
Footnotes, endnotes and list of references	[1] Graham Gibbs, *Learning by doing. A guide to teaching and learning methods.* Oxford: Oxford Polytechnic, Further Education Unit, 1988.

In author–date systems, sources in the list of references are organized alphabetically by surname, while in numerical systems they are organized numerically, in the order they appear in the text.

There are two basic ways of using references in your texts:

- in-text citation;
- quotation.

You use in-text citation when you borrow somebody else's ideas only, not their words. In-text citation acknowledges the source of ideas you are writing about in your own words. You can do this by:

- Adding references in brackets at the end of your own idea – for example, 'Reflection has been identified as an extremely useful skill for nurses (Durgahee 1996; Johns 1996; Mountford & Rogers 1996)'.
- Mentioning the author(s) and paraphrasing their ideas in your own words – for example, 'Allen (1990) suggests that patients...'

It is important to notice that there is a slight difference in emphasis between these two ways of using in-text citations. In the first case, where you use parenthetical references, the emphasis is on the ideas or contributions made by the author or authors. In the second, you emphasize the author's or authors' importance. This difference in emphasis is important, as you may sometimes need to specify the contribution made to the field by a specific person. For example, in most sources about reflection you will read 'Gibbs (1988)', as his name is associated with the development of reflective practice in nursing.

When you borrow not only other people's ideas – acknowledged by citation – but also their words, you are using quotation. Quoted text must be included between quotation marks ('like this text') to indicate that these are the exact words of the original text. Quotation marks also serve the purpose of separating your own words from those of other people. This is a basic tool to help you avoid plagiarism (also see Chapter 9).

In the case of quotations, you must provide:

- The surname(s) of the author(s).
- The year of the publication.
- The page number(s) of the original text.

In summary, you need to reference when you:

- Borrow ideas or information from other sources.
- Quote somebody's words and ideas exactly as they were in the original text.
- Paraphrase somebody's ideas in your own words.
- Summarize somebody's ideas in your own words.
- Reproduce a graph, table or diagram from another source.

The way in which you organize these pieces of information will vary depending on the referencing system you need to follow. In nursing and midwifery, the most commonly used systems of referencing are the Harvard system and the American Psychological Association (APA) style. The Vancouver system is also used, though less commonly. We will examine these three systems in more detail in the next sections.

The Harvard system

The Harvard system is a popular method of referencing in higher education although there is no single version of the system and each version varies slightly. It is, however, the most commonly used system in nursing and midwifery studies and in the following tables you will find the most usual conventions for referencing sources following this system. Conventions for in-text citations and quotations are listed in Tables 10.6 and 10.7, while conventions for lists of references are given in Table 10.8.

Table 10.6 Conventions for in-text citations using the Harvard system		
Convention	Avoid	Example
In-text citations should include the author's or authors' surnames (up to three authors), followed by the year of publication.	Using first names or first-name initials.	This has been identified as a central issue in contemporary health care (Perry, 2004).
Use 'and' for sources by more than one author.	Avoid using ampersand (&)	The potential causes of maternal postnatal concern and distress have been examined from different perspectives (Littlewood and McHugh, 1997).
When paraphrasing other people's ideas, use their surname(s), followed by the year of publication in round brackets.	Using ampersand (&) between the authors' surnames	Potter and Perry (2004) have identified it as a central issue in contemporary health care.

Convention	Avoid	Example
When you cite more than one source, you should organize them in chronological order.	Organizing sources in alphabetical order.	This view has been supported by a number of practitioners (Roberts, 2000; Brown, 2001; Allen, 2002).
Use the phrase 'as cited in' followed by the source details when you are quoting something already quoted in your source. Include both sources in the list of references.	Quoting the secondary source as if you had read it.	Smith (1999, as cited in Clark 2004, p. 121) supported the idea of a new approach to nurse education that would include a strong reflective element.
Use '*et al.*' ('and others') for a source that has more than three authors the second time you mention the work. Use *italics* for this abbreviation.	Using a full stop after 'et'. It is a complete word. It is Latin for 'and'. Using '*et al.*' the first time you mention the work.	New approaches to woman care tend to place both the woman and the midwife at the centre of the care (Pairman *et al.* 2006).

Table 10.7 Conventions for quotations using the Harvard system

Convention	Avoid	Example
Use page numbers only if you reproduce (e.g. quote, paraphrase or summarize) information from another source.	Using a colon between year and page. Instead use a comma after the year and 'p.' before the page number. In case of two or more pages, use 'pp'.	However, as Page (2000, p. 10) points out, 'women having home births are well educated and healthy, and this may be a major factor influencing the outcomes of such studies'.
Quotations that are longer than two or three lines should be separated from the main text, indented and single spaced and put into a smaller font.	Using quotation marks for longer quotes.	Your text your text your text your text your text

Long quote long quote long quote long quote long quote

Your text your text your text your text. |
| Quotations from internet resources with no pagination should mention the paragraph number or line in the original text. | Paginating the web-based source yourself. | Stark (2004, line 34) claims that 'these areas of concern have tended to go unnoticed in most research to date'. |
| If no date is given in the source (e.g. a pamphlet), write 'no date'. | Using the abbreviation 'n.d.' for 'no date'. | This is a crucial step in educating the new mother (Enfield Health Centre, no date). |

Convention	Avoid	Example
Use the title of a source if you can't identify its author(s). This also applies to work published by a group organization.	Using 'anonymous' for newspapers or other popular sources.	The health and well-being of the aging population is a growing concern that requires intelligent and innovative responses (*Our health, our care, our say*, 2006).
For an article without an author (e.g. newspaper), use the name of the publication instead.		Overseas nurses in the UK have encountered problems for being promoted to better, more challenging positions (*The Guardian*, 2005).

Table 10.8 Conventions for lists of references using the Harvard system

Convention	Avoid	Example
References should be alphabetically organized.	Using bullets or numbers for the sources in your list.	Courtenay, M. (2002)... Godin, P. (2003a)... Godin, P. (2003b)... Warne, T. and McAndrew, S. (2004) ...
Use *italics* for the title of books and name of journals. Capitalize only the first word of a book title.	Using italics for the title of chapters in books and articles in journals.	Warne, T. and McAndrew, S. (2004) *Using patient experience in nurse education*. Basingstoke: Palgrave.
The author's surname should be followed by a comma and the author's name initial or initials, followed by the year of publication in round brackets.	Using square brackets for the year of publication.	Jasper, M. (2003) *Beginning reflective practice: Foundations in nursing and health care*. Cheltenham: Nelson Thornes.
Titles of chapters and articles should be enclosed in single quotes and only their first word capitalized. Page numbers should also be given.	Using double quotation marks ("text").	Courtenay, M. (2002). 'Movement and mobility', in Hogston, R. and Simpson, P. M. (eds.) *Foundations of nursing practice*. Basingstoke: Palgrave, pp. 262–85.
Include the edition of a book only if it is **not** the first.	Using 'ed' to abbreviate edition. Use 'edn' instead. Sometimes 'e' is used as in '2e' (second edition), but this has not become an established convention yet.	Johnson, T. and Taylor, W. (2005) *Skills for midwifery practice*. 2nd edn. London: Churchill Livingstone.

Convention	Avoid	Example
Internet resources (e.g. webpages) should contain the complete URL (uniform resource locator) and the date they were last accessed.		Standards of proficiency for nurse and midwife prescribers. NMC (2005). Available at: https://www.nmc.org.uk/ standards/additional-standards/ standards-of-proficiency-for-nurse-and-midwife-prescribers/ (Accessed: 23 March 2018).
Use letters (a, b, c) after the year for multiple publications by the same author(s) in the same year.		Godin, P. (2003a) 'Class inequalities in mental health nursing', in Miers, M. (ed.) *Class inequalities and nursing practice.* Basingstoke: Palgrave, pp. 125–43.
		Godin, P. (2003b) 'The frontline workforce of community mental health care', in Hannigan, B. and Coffey, M. (eds.) *The handbook of community mental health nursing.* London: Routledge, pp. 19–29.
		Godin, P. (2003c) 'Be very afraid', *Mental health nursing*, 23(3), pp. 12–13.
Include the editor's or editors' names in edited collections.	Using '(Ed.)' for volumes that have been edited by more than one editor. Use '(Eds.)' instead.	Courtenay, M. (2002) 'Movement and mobility' in Hogston, R. and Simpson, P. M. (Eds.) *Foundations of nursing practice.* Basingstoke: Palgrave, pp. 262–85.

ACTIVITY 10.3

Based on what you have learnt about in-text citations and quotations following the Harvard system, read this text and identify what is wrong with each reference.

Dual-diagnosis specialists are becoming increasingly aware of the need to develop a treatment model that addresses the challenges posed by clients with severe mental health problems and a history of misuse substances (Philips P. & Joanne Labrow 1998). There are a few intervention programmes to treat clients with a dual diagnosis. However, they are relatively new and have not been objectively evaluated for their effectiveness (Rassool 2001, pp. 110). In some countries, increasing attention to these issues is being paid and, as a result, several integrated-approach treatment programmes have been set up. These involve specialized multidisciplinary teams, working to address the unmet needs of clients (www.mind.org.uk). This essay will briefly describe the existing models, and thoroughly examine their value. Against this background, the essay will evaluate the potentials of the new programmes in the light of the results obtained in their implementation.

Answers See suggested answers on p. 205.

The APA style

The American Psychological Association (APA) style is also an author–date system that is sometimes recommended by some nursing and midwifery lecturers. However, it is more common in publications such as professional journals.

In Tables 10.9 and 10.10 you will find the most common conventions for referencing sources following the APA style that differ from the ones given by the Harvard style.

Table 10.9   Conventions for in-text citations and quotations using the APA style

Convention	Avoid	Example
In-text citations should include the author's or authors' surnames (up to six), followed by a comma, followed by the year of publication.	Using first names or first-name initials.	This has been identified as a central issue in contemporary health care (Potter & Perry, 2004).
When you cite more than one source, organize them alphabetically and separate them with a semicolon.	Organizing sources chronologically.	This view has been supported by many practitioners (Allen, 2002; Brown, 2001; Roberts, 2000).
The first time you use a source with up to six authors, use all surnames. Use the first author's surname followed by 'et al.' ('and others') for more than six authors and for subsequent citations of the source. Use *italics* for this abbreviation.	Using a full stop after 'et'.	Care for the pregnant woman has been a crucial issue in midwifery (Pairman, Pincombe, Thorogood & Tracy, 2006). New approaches to woman care tend to place both the woman and the midwife at the centre of the care (Pairman *et al.*, 2006).
Use ampersand (&) for more than one author in in-text citation.	Using ampersand (&) when the author(s) are not within brackets.	The potential causes of maternal postnatal concern and distress have been examined from different perspectives (Littlewood & McHugh, 1997).

Table 10.10   Conventions for lists of references using the APA style

Convention	Avoid	Example
The author's surname should be followed by a comma and the author's name initial or initials, followed by the year of publication between round brackets.		Jasper, M. (2003). *Beginning reflective practice: Foundations in nursing and health care.* Cheltenham: Nelson Thornes.

Convention	Avoid	Example
Titles of book chapters should *not* be enclosed in quotes and only their first word should be capitalized. Page numbers should appear in round brackets right after the title of the book.		Courtenay, M. (2002). Movement and mobility, in R. Hogston & P.M. Simpson (Eds.), *Foundations of nursing practice* (pp. 262–85). Basingstoke: Palgrave.
For journal articles, use italics for the name of the journal, followed by a comma, followed by the volume number, followed by a colon and the page numbers.	Using the abbreviation 'pp.' for the page numbers, and round brackets.	Fine, M.A. & Kurdek, L.A. (1993). Reflections on determining authorship credit and authorship order on faculty-student collaborations. *American Psychologist*, 48: 1141–47.

ACTIVITY 10.4

Based on what you have learnt about lists of references following the APA style, read this text and spot any errors or omissions.

Courtenay, M. 2002. Movement and mobility in R. Hogston & P.M. Simpson (Eds.): *Foundations of nursing practice*, 262–85. Basingstoke: Palgrave.
Johnson, T. and W. Taylor. (2005). *Skills for midwifery practice*. Second edn. London: Churchill Livingstone.
Jasper, M. (2003). *Beginning reflective practice: Foundations in nursing and health care*. Cheltenham: Nelson Thornes.
Savage, T.A. (2005). How do we handle conflicts with parents over unsafe oral feedings? *Rehabilitation Nursing*, 30, (pp. 7–8).

Answers See suggested answers on p. 205.

The Vancouver system

The Vancouver system is a numerical system. In a numerical system a number is assigned to each reference as it appears in the text. This number becomes the 'unique identifier' of that reference and it is used each time that reference is cited. In other words, the first reference you cite will be numbered [1] in the text, and the second reference you cite will be numbered [2]. When you cite reference number 1 again, you will cite it using the number [1]. Even when the name of the author appears in your text, it should be followed by the number of the reference.

Let us look at an example. This same example appeared on p. 000 but following the Harvard system of referencing. You may wish to compare both examples and see how a numerical and an author–date system differ. The main conventions for Vancouver in-text citations, quotations and references are listed in Tables 10.11, 10.12 and 10.13.

The differences seen are not explainable by disappointment with the care-giver assignment. Staniszewska and Ahmed [1] point out that patients' expectations are influenced by their awareness of what they realistically expect. Evaluation of a service is also influenced by beliefs about the duty the service owes the client and whether or not there were circumstances outside the service's control that affected the care. [2] If expectations are a determinant of satisfaction with care, there is then less difference between the satisfaction scores of the two groups since women have different expectations for doctors than they do for midwives. (Adapted from Harvey *et al.* 2002, p. 266)

Table 10.11   Main in-text conventions for the Vancouver system

Convention	Example
Numbers are inserted to the right of commas and full stops, and to the left of colons and semicolons.	This has been identified as a central issue in contemporary health care. [1]
Multiple sources can be listed at a single reference point. The numbers are then separated by commas and consecutive numbers are joined with a dash.	The potential causes of maternal postnatal concern and distress have been examined from different perspectives. [2–6, 11, 21]

Table 10.12   Main quotation conventions for the Vancouver system

Convention	Example
Use double quotation marks to enclose a direct quotation.	However, as Page points out, "women having home births are well educated and healthy, and this may be a major factor influencing the outcomes of such studies." [3]
Quotations that are longer than two or three lines should be separated from the main text, indented and single spaced and put into a smaller font.	Your text your text your text your text your text [4] Long quote long quote long quote long quote long quote Your text your text your text your text.

Table 10.13 List of reference conventions for the Vancouver system

Convention	Example
The reference list is arranged numerically in the order in which references are cited in the text.	[1] M. Courtenay.... [2] P. Godin..... [3] T. Warne & S. McAndrew. ... [4] P. Allen....
Use normal font for the title of books and name of journals. Capitalize only their first word and proper names.	T. Warne & S. McAndrew. Using patient experience in nurse education. Basingstoke: Palgrave; 2004.
The author's surname should follow the author's name initial. A full stop should follow.	M. Jasper
Authors' names should be followed by the title of the book or journal article preceded by a comma. A full stop should follow.	Beginning reflective practice: Foundations in nursing and health care.
The title of the book should be followed by the place of publication, followed by a colon, and then followed by the publishing house. A semicolon should follow. Finally the year of publication should be added.	Cheltenham: Nelson Thornes; 2003.
In the case of a journal article, the title of the article should be followed by the abbreviated name of the journal, followed by the year of publication, followed by a semicolon, followed by the volume and issue number, followed by a colon, followed by the page numbers.	N. Wharton. Health and safety in outdoor activity centres. J Adventure Ed Outdoor Lead. 1996; 12(4):8–9.
Journal titles are abbreviated. A list of abbreviations for the titles is available from PubMed at www.ncbi. nlm.nih.gov/journals. To view the abbreviated form of a journal title, enter the full journal title in the search box at the top.	Some examples of journal abbreviations: Pract Midwife: The Practising Midwife; Nurs Stand: Nursing Standard; Nurs Ethics: Nursing Ethics; Community Pract: Community Practitioner; J Adv Nurs: Journal of Advanced Nursing.

Engaging with sources: Working with other people's texts

Reporting verbs

In academic writing **reporting verbs** can be used to:

- **report** on a previous experiment or study,
- **discuss** other people's ideas, views or beliefs, and
- **describe** previous research activities or methods.

The verb a writer chooses to introduce either a quote or a paraphrase (see Chapter 9) indicates the relationship between the writer and the text he/she is quoting. Thus, different reporting verbs will indicate a different relationship or function (e.g. to report on a previous experiment, to discuss an idea).

So, when choosing which reporting verb to use to introduce a quote or paraphrase, you have to first decide what function or relationship you want to establish. Table 10.14 shows the main functions of key reporting verbs.

Table 10.14 Functions of frequently used reporting verbs

Function	Typical verbs	Example
To report on a previous experiment or study	analyse, explore, emphasize, notice, observe, point out, state, write	Brown (2013) **observes** that further studies are needed to gather conclusive evidence.
To discuss other people's ideas, views or beliefs	argue, believe, claim, conceptualize, conclude, consider, criticize, focus on, hold, prefer, note, reiterate	They **claim** that hospital staff need a high level of mobility because they must reach other persons or places and access a variety of resources on a daily basis.
To describe previous research activities or methods	conclude, describe, discover, discuss, find, find out, identify, obtain, report, show	In their latest study, Collins *et al.* (2016) **discussed** the benefits of early interventions for this type of patient.

ACTIVITY 10.5

Let's now look at some pairs of sentences that illustrate the key functions of reporting verbs. As you read the pairs, think of what the underlined words tell you about the relationship between the writer and the reported texts or ideas.

Pair 1

1.1 Their study provides an analysis of the time nurses in surgical units spend with patients and other staff.

1.2 Their study claims that the time nurses in surgical units spend with patients and other staff is of crucial importance.

Pair 2

2.1 Jenkins *et al.* (2014) found a high degree of discrepancy among the results presented in the 23 empirical studies they examined.

2.2　Jenkins *et al.* (2014) strongly criticized the high degree of discrepancy among the results presented in the 23 empirical studies they examined.

Pair 3

3.1　In various sections of the study, the author repeats the idea that previous hypotheses have failed to statistically demonstrate the existence of such a link.

3.2　In various sections of the study, the author reiterates the idea that previous hypotheses have failed to statistically demonstrate the existence of such a link.

Answers See suggested answers on p. 206.

ACTIVITY 10.6

Read the following sentences and match them with one of the purposes described in the labels provided below. The first one has been done as an example.

(A) To report on a previous experiment or study	(B) To discuss other people's ideas, views or beliefs	(c) To describe previous re-search activities or methods

Examples	Function
1. In their review of studies on the contributions of community nursing to Scottish people's health, Kennedy and her colleagues (2008) examined 12 systematic reviews and 61 studies and concluded that, given the proper support, community nurses are in an ideal place to anticipate and help prevent health problems.	C
2. Crowe *et al.* (2016) observed that despite their condition many patients who experience multimorbidity are capable of self-managing their health successfully if they are supported appropriately.	
3. As a result of their systematic review, Phillippi, Danhausen, Alliman and Phillippi (2018) concluded that the flaws in the literature on the effect of birth centre care on neonatal outcomes are rather substantial and therefore more research is needed to address the situation.	

4. The study followed women for five years after they requested an abortion at 30 different facilities across the USA. Participants for the study were recruited between January 2008 and December 2010.

5. Their pilot study demonstrated that interventions that included mindfulness and skills-based childbirth education would help pregnant women to develop greater confidence in giving birth.

Answers See suggested answers on p. 206.

Reporting verbs and text sections

Some reporting verbs are more frequently associated with a particular section of the text being reported. For example, 'examine' (e.g. 'The study examined a number of...') is usually used to indicate the 'aims' of the study, whereas 'show' often refers to its 'results' (e.g. 'The results of the study show that...'). Table 10.15 provides examples of reporting verbs most commonly associated with the different sections of a journal article.

Table 10.15 Reporting verbs and text sections		
Section of article	Reporting verb	Example
Aim (in the introduction)	aim, analyse, be concerned with, examine, consider, investigate, identify, focus on, look at, report	Their study **is concerned with** identifying the key factors affecting obesity.
Methods	collect, conduct, incorporate, interview, undertake	O'Sullivan (2015) **incorporated** 30 studies published in the five journals between 2010 and 2014.
Results	confirm, find, identify, indicate, suggest, reveal, show	Their findings **reveal** that the correlation between the two variables is higher if socio-economic factors are taken into account.
Discussion	indicate, offer, provide	Kimberly's (2001) discussion **offers** further support.
Conclusion	conclude	O'Sullivan (2015) **concluded** that more research in this area is needed.

Tenses for reporting verbs

Tenses are another important element to consider when we quote or paraphrase. The most frequent tenses used to report other people's work, ideas or beliefs are:

- **The simple present** (e.g. 'They **report** a number of...', 'The evidence **shows** that...')
- **The simple past** (e.g. 'They **surveyed** a sample of...', 'Alderson (2012) **brought** two...')
- **The present perfect** (e.g. 'Several studies **have emphasized** that...')

Very often reporting verbs are used in **the present tense** (e.g. 'Smith (2015) **seems** to subscribe to early theories') in order to give emphasis to what is being reported, that is, 'to bring past research into the present'. This is particularly the case when what you report refers to **facts** or **theories**, as the following example shows:

1 Their study **challenges** the doctrine of patient-centred care delivery models that largely **focus** on wait times for surgical interventions.

However, when reporting verbs refer to processes and procedures (as in the methods section of a journal article), the **simple past** is preferred.

2 In their recent study Brown and colleagues (2015) **considered** a number of variables affecting patients with the condition.

The **present perfect** is the most common tense for reporting verbs that

- introduce a topic by referring to the existing research in a particular area (see example 3 below);
- refer to what has been done so far in a particular field (see example 4 below),
- show a contrast between what has been done so far and what is lacking, often referred to as 'a gap in the literature' (see example 5 below).

3 A number of studies (e.g. Alexander 2001; Brown *et al.* 2015; Smith 2015) **have shown** how relational continuity in childbearing can influence the woman's birth experience.

4 In the existing literature (e.g. Kimberly 2001; Alexander *et al.* 2015; O'Sullivan 2015), this **has been claimed** to be a key area in midwifery care.

5 Although the topic was considered in a number of studies in the past ten years (e.g. Brown 2010; Jenkins *et al.* 2014; Collins *et al.* 2016), not all aspects relating to primigravida women **have received** meticulous attention.

Reporting verbs in nursing and midwifery

The following examples have been taken from published research in nursing and midwifery. For each example, can you identify:

- The function of the reporting verb (e.g. to report on a previous experiment);
- The tense that has been used (e.g. simple present) and
- The reason why that particular tense was chosen (e.g. to give emphasis)?

ACTIVITY 10.7

Examples	Function	Tense	Reason for choice of tense
1. Crowe *et al.* (2016) <u>have argued</u> that improving the care of older people who suffer from multimorbidity is a considerable challenge for most health-care systems worldwide.			
2. In their 2009 study, they <u>tested</u> the internal consistency and reliability of their data-collection instruments on a group of 46 subjects.			
3. Based on the results of their study, they <u>concluded</u> that improved self-efficacy of birthing women could help them deal with previous psychological trauma of giving birth and lower their psychological and physiological stress.			
4. Shaw (2015) <u>has pointed out</u> that caring support from early stages of pregnancy in midwifery services is the most effective way of providing women with a positive birth experience.			
5. His study <u>demonstrated</u> statistically significant effect sizes and improvements in fitness and physical activity of the subjects in the experimental group.			
6. Using purposive sampling techniques, 25 research participants <u>were chosen</u> from the list ensuring diversity to take part in the focus groups.			
7. Thomson and Downe (2010) <u>highlight</u> that a strong connection between the birthing woman and the midwife <u>is</u> a simple but effective way to achieve a positive birth experience.			
8. Allgood and Kvalsund (2005) <u>have indicated</u> that predictability <u>is linked</u> to a more mature phase in the relationship where mutual dependence is developed.			

Answers See suggested answers on p. 207.

Bibliographical software programs

Bibliographic software programs are packages that can help you organize your references. They are relatively easy to use and more and more universities are adopting them. They contain most referencing styles (both author–date and numerical systems) and you can change styles once you have created your own library of references.

In this section, you will find a short description and some examples of two of these software programs: EndNote and RefWorks.

EndNote

EndNote is a tool designed to help you manage your references, among other things. (A free trial of EndNote can be downloaded from http://endnote.com/downloads/30-day-trial. (Last accessed on 23 March 2018.)) With EndNote you can:

- Search bibliographical databases on the internet.
- Organize references and images in a database.
- Create your own library of references.
- Add a new reference, or change or delete it.
- Construct your paper with built-in manuscript templates.
- Watch the bibliography and figure list appear as you write.

Because EndNote works in a Windows environment, it will be easy for you to use it if you are familiar with any Windows word processor.

Adding a new reference is done by type (e.g. journal article, book, conference proceedings etc.) and you do not need to worry about formatting (capitals, font type etc.) as EndNote will do it for you according to the style you select. The template for adding new data, called a blank data entry screen, is shown in Figure 10.1. The window for managing the data you entered should look like Figure 10.2.

Figure 10.1 A blank EndNote data entry screen

Figure 10.2 An EndNote managing data window

Figure 10.1 shows the form that you use to enter your data. You have different fields for entering information and you don't need to worry about how to organize these fields as EndNote will do it for you.

Once you have created your own library using the form shown in Figure 10.1, you can manage the references within it. As Figure 10.2 illustrates, in the managing data window you can see the list of references in the library you have created. You can highlight one reference and see the complete notes you made for it; and you can decide to see the list by author, year or title.

Another very interesting facility that EndNote offers is the possibility of inserting references in your paper as you write. This facility is called 'cite while you write' (CWYW). For this, you need to access EndNote from the 'Tools' dropdown menu of your word processor. This menu enables you to use EndNote within your word processor document. You will also have an EndNote toolbar from which you can find a reference you require, insert it into your document and choose the style you need your references to observe. EndNote includes more than 1300 bibliographical styles. An EndNote screen for 'cite while you write' should look like Figure 10.3.

Figure 10.3 An EndNote CWYW screen

RefWorks

RefWorks is web-based software for managing bibliographies. (A free trial of RefWorks can be requested at www.proquest.com/products-services/refworks.html. (Last accessed on 23 March 2018.)) This means that you can access it from any internet-connected computer or laptop. It requires no special software and is automatically upgraded. RefWorks allows you to import references from different sources, organize them and easily manage them in folders.

RefWorks also allows you to format your references (for both in-text citations and the list of references) in more than 500 styles. Added to this, the package enables you to create your own style of referencing. RefWorks works in a Windows, Mac or Linux environment and it should be very simple for you to become familiar with it if you know how to use a word processor. The RefWorks window for importing references should look like the screenshot shown in Figure 10.4.

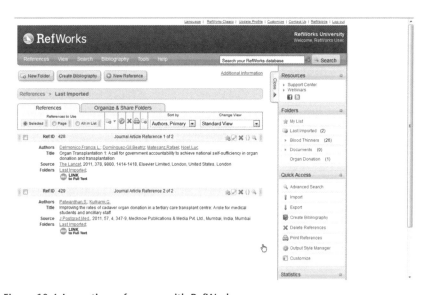

Figure 10.4 Importing references with RefWorks

RefWorks also features a 'write and cite' function that you can use for adding references to your work as you write it. This is simply done by using the function 'insert' in your word processor. A window for defining the output style format – that is, whether you want to use the Harvard or the APA system, for instance – looks as shown in Figure 10.5.

Figure 10.5 Defining the output style in RefWorks

Free bibliographical software programs

Zotero: www.zotero.org (Last accessed on 23 March 2018)
Zotero is a free tool that helps you

- collect;
- organize;
- cite;
- synchronize; and
- share sources.

Zotero **collects** research files in a single, searchable interface. Files such as PDFs, images, audio and video files and snapshots of webpages can be easily added and automatically indexed, enabling you to find exactly what you're looking for.

Zotero also **organizes** files into collections, similarly to how music playlists are organized. New items can be then added to any named collections.

Zotero allows you to **cite** by creating footnotes, endnotes, in-text citations, or bibliographies. You can create citations in 'Word' and 'OpenOffice' and add references to an email, a 'Google Doc', or other editors.

Zotero automatically **synchronizes** data across devices, and allows you to **share** your research library, complete with files, bibliographic data, notes, and discussion threads with another researcher or a research group.

WIKINDX http://wikindx.sourceforge.net (Last accessed on 23 March 2018)
WIKINDX is a Virtual Research Environment (an online bibliographic and quotations/notes management and article authoring system) designed either for

single use (on a variety of operating systems) or multi-user collaborative use across the internet.

Refbase www.refbase.net/index.php/Web_Reference_Database (Last accessed on 23 March 2018)

Refbase is a web-based, platform-independent, multi-user interface for managing scientific literature and citations. Figure 10.6 shows a screenshot of the main page.

Figure 10.6 **Screenshot of Refbase main page**

Revising the objectives of this chapter

Tick those objectives that you feel you have achieved and review those you have not yet managed to accomplish. Then, complete the **Achievement Chart** at the back of the book.

In this chapter, you have learnt to:

☐ recognize the basic principles of referencing

☐ identify the main referencing conventions of the Harvard, the APA and the Vancouver systems

☐ engage with sources

☐ recognize the basic uses of bibliographical software programs.

LIBRARY, UNIVERSITY OF CHESTER

Conclusion: Putting It All Together

Like any other type of writing, academic writing is best approached as a **process** and a **product**. The process starts with an examination of the question your assignment has to answer and a consideration of the most effective ways to answer it. It then moves on to gathering relevant information and to organizing and structuring this information in blocks. However, more often than not when structuring information you will probably need to go back to planning so as to reorganize the information in the most effective way. Once you have written your first draft, you will need to become an editor of your product. Editing your work requires a combination of macro abilities that you use in the writing process to look at the organization and structuring of information, and micro skills that you need to look at sentence structure and punctuation, for instance.

The chapters in this book have been arranged in three parts, which examine both the process and the product of writing. In the first part, you covered the **essentials of academic writing**: examining assignment questions, gathering information, and organizing and structuring the information into paragraphs, and paragraphs into essays. You also explored the differences between descriptive and argumentative writing, and examined typical genres that require these types of writing: the care critique, the journal article review and the argumentative essay. You finally analysed two essential processes that form the basis for many of these academic genres: reflection and critical thinking.

In the second part of the book you learnt **how to write in specific genres** in nursing and midwifery. The first chapter in this part elaborated on the foundations laid in the previous part and examined how to write a reflective essay. Then you moved on to analyse a more analytical genre: the care critique. You explored planning and organizing principles in writing a care critique, and learnt to structure it more effectively as well as to make sensible recommendations. Next, you learnt how to write argumentative texts and looked at three essential elements in argumentation: the strength of an argument, its structure and its language. The last chapter in this second part introduced you to the basis of writing in other typical genres in nursing and midwifery: action plans, care plans, portfolios, reports and research proposals. It also showed the preliminary steps you need to take when preparing to write your undergraduate dissertation.

The first two parts dealt with academic writing as a process. The last part approached writing as a product, giving you the basic tools to become the editor of your own work. In this last part, you learnt to **work with texts**. You learnt how to add variety to your texts, how to make them more cohesive, and you looked into what we call 'good writing style'. Coupled with this, in this part you dealt with plagiarism and learnt how to reference sources correctly following an author–date or a numerical referencing system.

It is important for you to see writing as both a **process** and a **product**. As a process, writing means drafting and redrafting. Even the most accomplished writers need to draft and redraft, moving from planning to structuring, only to go back to planning again. For the product of writing, you need to learn to become an editor of your own work, distancing yourself from it and using the marking criteria for the assignment you are writing to make sure that your 'product' meets the demands of the task at hand. To this end, you can use the different checklists in the chapters of this book to help you edit your work. More importantly, use the book's checklists as the basis on which to design your own.

We started this book with the idea that academic writing is one of the most difficult tasks we encounter when we start university. As with all other academic tasks, academic writing is a skill that can be learnt and perfected with dedication and practice. I hope that now you have reached the end of the book you will feel more confident about writing your assignments. You have covered all the necessary theoretical background you need to know to be able to write effectively, and you have also done exercises that have illustrated the main theoretical principles. Now you are ready to put it all together: to put theory into practice!

ACHIEVEMENT CHART

Use this chart to plot your achievements. If you have not achieved an objective (✗) or you are not sure about it (?), plan some action that will contribute to its achievement, for example revise the corresponding section in the book or ask your personal or support tutor for guidance.

Unit	Objectives	Achieved ✓/✗/?	Action to take
1	▶ Recognize the five basic principles of planning in academic writing.		
	▶ Identify the three elements in essay questions and follow marking criteria.		
	▶ Understand gathering, organizing and structuring information.		
	▶ Reproduce the generic structure of academic texts.		
	▶ Identify the main problems with sentence fragments, cohesion, dangling modifiers and punctuation.		
2	▶ Recognize the difference between description and argumentation.		
	▶ Identify the main academic genres in nursing and midwifery.		
	▶ Understand the purpose and the structure of these academic genres.		
	▶ Identify the main language items used in descriptive and critical writing.		
3	▶ Recognize the nature and stages of the reflective process.		
	▶ Identify different critical thinking processes.		
	▶ Understand the principles of the critical evaluation of evidence.		
	▶ Identify the key language items used in reflective and critical writing.		

Unit	Objectives	Achieved √ / x /?	Action to take
4	▶ Plan a reflective essay appropriately.		
	▶ Identify an effective way of introducing reflective essays.		
	▶ Recognize the structure of body paragraphs to support introductions.		
	▶ Recognize ways of producing an effective conclusion.		
	▶ Write effective reflective accounts of performance.		
	▶ Identify the style of the reflective essay.		
5	▶ Define the care critique.		
	▶ Plan and organize the care critique effectively.		
	▶ Structure the main sections of the care critique.		
	▶ Provide effective conclusions and make sensible recommendations.		
6	▶ Recognize the difference between opinion and argumentation.		
	▶ Identify the strength of an argument.		
	▶ Structure arguments effectively.		
	▶ Identify the main language items used in argumentative writing.		
7	▶ Write action plans.		
	▶ Write care plans.		
	▶ Prepare, write and choose an appropriate format for portfolios.		
	▶ Use a personal diary template.		

Unit	Objectives	Achieved √/x/?	Action to take
	▶ Produce reports.		
	▶ Write systematic reviews.		
	▶ Respond to case studies.		
	▶ Identify effective ways of producing research proposals.		
	▶ Plan to start writing your dissertation.		
8	▶ Recognize different ways of adding variety to your texts.		
	▶ Identify different sentence openers.		
	▶ Use cohesive devices to support textual variety.		
	▶ Recognize the different structural elements used for adding variety between parts of a text.		
9	▶ Recognize what constitutes plagiarism and what does not.		
	▶ Deal with definitions and concepts already well established in your field.		
	▶ Paraphrase other people's ideas and words without plagiarizing.		
10	▶ Recognize the basic principles of referencing.		
	▶ Identify the main referencing conventions of the Harvard system.		
	▶ Identify the main referencing conventions of the APA system. (**10.3**)		
	▶ Identify the main referencing conventions of the Vancouver system.		
	▶ Engage with sources.		
	▶ Recognize the basic uses of bibliographical software programs.		

Glossary of Key Terms

Note: Words in **bold** have been defined elsewhere in the glossary. Numbers in brackets indicate the chapter that deals with the word/phrase being defined.

A

Analyse: To examine the structure or components of something in order to explain it. (7)

Appropriate: (In relation to evidence) the relevance and reliability of the evidence provided in support of an argument. (7)

Argumentative writing: Writing that aims at persuading the reader about the validity, importance or significance of a point made or stance taken by the writer. It uses evidence to support the claims made and usually makes recommendations. (2) (6)

Articles: There are three articles in English: 'a', 'an' (indefinite articles) and 'the' (definite article). (7)

Article review: A price of writing that evaluates an article published in an academic or professional journal. (2)

Assessment/marking criteria: A set of principles used to judge the value and contribution of a written piece. In academic writing the assessment or marking criteria for an assignment normally accompany the instructions for it. (1) (7)

B

Bibliography: The list of sources that have been consulted or used in preparation of an academic document. This is presented at the end of an academic document and organized alphabetically. (Cf. **list of references**) (1)

C

Care critique: A systematic, critical and impersonal analysis of the care provided to a patient. A care critique discusses the validity and evaluates the worth of the care. (2)

Claim: Something that is believed to be true and that is supported by evidence. (6)

Clinical scenario: A clinical scenario is a brief description of a clinical situation or event, used to improve the identification, assessment and treatment of health problems. (7)

Cohesion: What holds texts together. Cohesion is normally achieved by using connectives, related words or logical transitions. See also **logical relationships**. (1)

Critical analysis: Systematic, logical and impersonal examination of the contents included, the claims made and the sources of evidence used in an argument. (2)

Critical skills: Sets of abilities needed to examine and evaluate the worth and contribution of an argument, a piece of writing etc. (7)

186

E

Evidence-based: Evidence-based clinical or academic practice emphasizes the examination of evidence from research or reflection on clinical experience as the basis for decision making. It de-emphasizes intuition and unsystematic experience, and requires skills such as literature searching and critical evaluation of sources. (1)

F

Font size: The size of the font used in a document, measured in points. In academic documents, the common size is 11 or 12 pts. (1)

Font style: The type of font used in a document. In academic documents, the common font styles are Arial and Times New Roman. Fanciful fonts are normally avoided. (1)

G

Generic functions: The function that a part of a genre is supposed to fulfil. For example, one generic function that introductions are supposed to have is 'stating the purpose of the text'. (5)

Generic genre: A genre that can be used as the basis for producing other associated genres. For example, the academic essay can be said to be a generic genre on which the reflective essay can be structured. (2)

Genres: The word 'genre' comes from the French (originally Latin) word for 'kind' or 'class'. Genres can be said to constitute particular conventions of content and/or form (including structure and style). These conventions are shared by all the texts that belong to the same class or genre. Thus, all reflective essays, for example, will share certain conventions as to content and form. (2)

I

Identify: To spot something and be able to say what it is, based on its main features or distinctive qualities or characteristics. (1) (7)

L

List of references: List of all the sources cited in a text. The list is presented at the end of an academic document and organized alphabetically. Compare with **bibliography**. (1)

Logical relationships: Relationships between the ideas in a text that are emphasized by the use of 'connectives'. See also **cohesion**. (2) (8)

M

Marking criteria: Set of criteria or statements used to mark a piece of writing. (1)

Meaningful: Having a particular meaning or purpose in relation to something else that is being studied or investigated. (7)

N

Narrow down: To focus on main points by selection or reducing them in number. (1)

O

Outline: To give a brief description of main features or issues. (1) (7)

P

Paragraph: A group of related (in topic and focus) sentences that makes complete sense on its own. Paragraphs may be short or long; what is important about paragraphs is that they develop only one central idea. (1)

Paragraphing: Arranging and structuring information into paragraphs. (1)

Paraphrasing: Expressing the same ideas and content of an original text, but using different words and structural elements. (9)

Parentheses ( ): Punctuation marks used to add extra, parenthetical information that is not necessary to understand the main/central idea being expressed. For example, 'In this format, the items are arranged in the order specified above (with the exception of specialized entries)'. (1)

Plagiarism: Intellectual dishonesty by which someone claims that other people's ideas or texts are their own. Plagiarism is usually the result of ignorance or cultural differences. Some students ignore the rules for citation and quotation that are regulated by different **referencing** systems. In some cultures, 'copying' other people's intellectual property may be considered a 'compliment'. (8)

Punctuation marks: Punctuation marks are used to signal pause, emphasis, expansion or clarification. The most frequently used punctuation marks are the apostrophe, colon, comma, dash, hyphen, **parentheses**, quotation marks and semicolon. (1)

Q

Question words: Words used to ask questions, sometimes called 'wh' words: what, where, when, why, who. But also notice how, how often, how long. (1)

R

Rationale: The reasons that explain why a particular decision has been made, a course of action followed etc. (1)

Referencing: A system of rules for citing and quoting other people's intellectual property that helps writers to avoid committing **plagiarism**. There are a number of systems, the most frequent being the Harvard System, the American Psychology Association (APA) system and the Modern Language Association (MLA) system. (10)

Reflection: The process by which a past event or occurrence is revisited to evaluate, from the present perspective, what happened and how its negative effects can be avoided in the future. (4)

Rephrase: Say something again by using different words. See also **paraphrasing**. (1)

Review protocol: A review protocol is a document that sets out the reviewers' intentions with regard to the topic and the methods to be used in carrying out a proposed review. It puts forward inclusion, also sometimes exclusion, criteria for the data which will be considered for the review. (7)

Rigorous: Thorough and careful, and done systematically following a set of pre-determined rules. (7)

S

Signpost: A word, phrase or sentence that is used to indicate the direction that an argument or idea will take or follow. (1)

Stance: The position that the writer of a text adopts in relation to the text s/he is producing. Stance is normally created by the use of linguistic devices such as 'modal verbs' and 'adverbs'. (2)

Summarize: To give a brief statement of the main points, aspects or issues of something. (7)

Supporting evidence: Evidence or practice-based examples used to support a claim made. (1)

Synthesize: To compare critically different materials, ideas or arguments, highlighting similarities, differences and connections. (7)

T

Text flow: The way ideas connect with one another in a text. The logical flow between the ideas in a text is reinforced by formal elements such as connectives and lexis. See also cohesion. (1)

Tone down: Make the claims made less comprehensive, extreme or offensive. (6)

Transitions/transition markers: A word, phrase or sentence used to mark the transition between ideas or paragraphs in a text. Transition markers are used to reinforce the flow between parts of a text or between texts. (3) (4)

Further Readings and Resources

This list indicates books and websites that you can turn to if you want to expand on any of the main topics in this text.

Critical thinking
Cottrell, Stella. (2017). *Critical thinking skills: Developing effective analysis and argument.* 3rd edn. London: Palgrave.
Milan, Deanne. (2006). *Developing critical reading skills.* 7th edn. New York: McGraw-Hill.
Van Den Brinkbudgen, Roy. (2000). *Critical thinking for students: Learn the skills of critical assessment and effective argument.* 3rd edn. Oxford: How To Books.

Plagiarism
Johns, Julia & Sarah Keller. (2005). *Cite it right: The SourceAid guide to citation, research, and avoiding plagiarism.* Boston, MA: SourceAid, LLC.
Pears, Richard & Graham Shields. (2016). *Cite them right: The essential guide to referencing and plagiarism.* 10th edn. London: Palgrave.

Punctuation
Peck, John & Martin Coyle. (2012). *The student's guide to writing: Grammar, punctuation and spelling.* 3rd edn. Basingstoke: Palgrave Macmillan.
Peck, John & Martin Coyle. (2012). *Write it right: The secrets of effective writing.* Basingstoke: Palgrave Macmillan.

Resources
University of Ottawa Punctuation webpage. Available at http://arts.uottawa.ca/centredcriture/en/hypergrammar/punctuation. Last accessed on 15 June 2018.

Referencing
Greetham, Bryan. (2018). *How to write better essays.* 4th edn. London: Palgrave.
Williams, Kate & Davis, Mary. (2017). *Referencing and understanding plagiarism.* 2nd edn. London: Palgrave.

Working with tables, charts and graphs
Etherington, Sue. (2002). *Tables, charts and graphs.* London: Dorling Kindersley Publishers.
Smyth, T.R. (2004). *The principles of writing in psychology.* Basingstoke: Palgrave Macmillan.

General

Atkins, S. & K. Murphy. (1993). Reflection: A review of the literature. *Journal of Advanced Nursing*, 18, 1188–92.

Buzan, T. (1991). *The mind map book*. New York: Penguin.

Dahlberg, U. & I. Aune. (2013). The woman's birth experience – The effect of interpersonal relationships and continuity of care. *Midwifery*, 29, 407–15.

Dayenne van Schie, D., S. Castelein, J. van der Bijl, R. Meijburg, R., B. Stringer & B. van Meijel. (2016) Systematic review of self-management in patients with schizophrenia: Psychometric assessment of tools, levels of self-management and associated factors. *Journal of Advanced Nursing*, 72(11), 2598–611.

Mareno N. & J.J. Annesi. (2016). A statement synthesis of emotional eating and body size recognition: Advancing nursing science related to obesity research. *Journal of Advanced Nursing*, 72(5), 1023–29.

Norberg, A., E. Melin & K. Asplunda. (2003). Reactions to music, touch and object presentation in the final stage of dementia: An exploratory study. *International Journal of Nursing Studies*, 40, 473–79.

Tsaya, S.-T. & M.-L. Chen. (2003). Acupressure and quality of sleep in patients with end-stage renal disease – a randomized controlled trial. *International Journal of Nursing Studies*, 40, 1–7.

Tummers, G.E.R., G.G. van Merode & J.A. Landeweerd. (2002). The diversity of work: Differences, similarities and relationships concerning characteristics of the organisation, the work and psychological work reactions in intensive care and non-intensive care nursing. *International Journal of Nursing Studies*, 39, 841–55.

Suggested Answers to Activities

Chapter 1

The table below lists the verbs you will see most often used in essay questions. Write the meaning of each verb in your own words. You do not need to provide complete sentences; key words will do. Use a dictionary if you are not sure of the meanings. 'Argue' and 'discuss' have been completed for you as examples.

Verb	Definition	Additional information
Analyse	To examine the structure or components of something to explain it.	To separate into parts.
Argue	To give reasons why something is right or wrong, true or untrue.	To persuade people.
Classify	To sort into groups.	According to features.
Demonstrate	To show what something is like, or how it works.	Using evidence or examples.
Differentiate	To show the main differences between things.	Key features or qualities.
Discuss	To examine in detail, showing the different opinions or ideas about something.	Frequently confused with 'argue', but a more balanced response is required in 'discuss'.
Evaluate	To calculate or judge the value of something.	It may require personal views.
Examine	To consider something carefully.	Considering its structure, components etc.
Explain	To give the reasons why something is what it is, or happens the way it does.	To get a better understanding of it.
Identify	To spot something and be able to say what it is.	Main features or qualities.
Outline	To give a description of main features or issues.	Should be brief.
Produce	To show something for examination.	In order to achieve an outcome.

ACTIVITY 1.2

How would you organize and structure the scrambled ideas to write an essay on this question? Here is one possibility. There may be others, but it's important that you realize that the list presents positive as well as negative aspects of communication in nursing.

The importance of effective communication in nursing

Positive
- Communication as a therapeutic space
- Collaboration and negotiation skills with clients and families
- Facilitating empathy

Negative
- Common barriers to effective communication
- Dealing with aggression

ACTIVITY 1.3

The paragraph has five sentences. Can you identify

1 The sentence that introduces the general idea of the text (**topic**)?
    Nurses can work in many health-care settings, which gives them the opportunity to gain experience in all aspects of caring for clients and their families.

2 Another sentence that provides the focus/point of view of the topic (**focus**)?
    Nurses can thus build their professional career in many different ways.

3 The examples that develop/support the focus (**examples/evidence**)?
    They may choose to become clinical specialists or consultant nurses, or they can opt for managerial positions as a head of nursing services or supervisor of other nurses. Some may prefer to pursue an academic career in education and research.

4 The sentence that brings the text to an end (**conclusion**)?
    These are just a few examples of the opportunities that nurses currently have to develop their professional interests.

Chapter 2

ACTIVITY 2.1

Essay question 1
What does providing care for the critically ill patient involve? Discuss.

Introduction 1
It provides a good start with a clear topic and focus. However, it doesn't include much more than that. It doesn't say how the essay will be developed, and it is very difficult to anticipate what you will find in it.

Essay question 2
Analyse the role of reassurance in nursing care.

Introduction 2
This is the very start of an introduction. It clearly identifies the topic and the focus. It organizes information from general to specific and provides enough information to convey the point it is trying to make.

It also includes a short description of what the essay will do. It is, however, a little incomplete as it does not mention everything the essay will do, which you expect after the connective 'first'.

Essay question 3
Evaluate the value of models for treating dual-diagnosis clients.

Introduction 3
This is a very good and complete introduction. It has a clear topic and focus. It includes enough information for the reader to know what it is going to be about. It also states how the essay will develop its topic and its focus.

ACTIVITY 2.2

This is a very effective outline (1). It covers all points related to the essay question and shows that the writer is aware of the marking criteria, especially criteria 2, 3 and 4, and knows how to use them to plan the critique. It also shows a balance between theory and practice and plans to incorporate the writer's experience on clinical placement.

ACTIVITY 2.3

This is a good example of an introduction of an article review. It states both the topic of the article and the purpose of the review. It also mentions the audience of the article and the assumptions the writer has made about them. It describes the journal as an appropriate forum for the article, which is described as an empirical article. However, there is no information about the journal volume and issue, and no page numbers for the article.

ACTIVITY 2.5

Text 2 is more descriptive. It just presents a list of facts: having to make decisions, benefits of staying in the same room, locations of nurses' stations and patient privacy. In contrast, **Text 1** is more argumentative. It provides a balanced view of the topic by presenting arguments in favour of returning a patient with a stroke to the open-plan unit as well as those in support of allowing the patient to stay in the same room.

Chapter 3

ACTIVITY 3.2

The writer positions him/herself as an objective outsider, focusing on the studies and programmes and their results. S/he agrees with some aspects of the studies mentioned but also indicates some of their shortcomings (e.g. 'This seems to indicate that smoking cessation in pregnancy is unsuccessful because ...'). The writer uses a variety of verbs to indicate endorsement or the lack of it (e.g. 'suggest', 'seem to', 'forcefully concluded', 'should'). S/he presents the arguments that will later be challenged, but doesn't provide a transition such as 'however'. Instead, there is a suggestion that these studies indicate that support has been unsuccessful.

In this part of the text, the writer refers to previous arguments on which the new arguments are built. However, no new evidence to support his/her points is being presented. Nevertheless, it is difficult to judge at this point the balance in the arguments as well as the logical relationship between the different parts of the argument.

The presentation of the arguments follows a logical order and this helps with the writer's aim to convince the reader, but it may be, again, too early to say.

ACTIVITY 3.3

1 Maslin-Prothero is affiliated with a university in the UK, has edited several books and is a regular contributor to various journals. The text is published in association with the Royal College of Nursing in the UK. It was edited some years ago, but a second edition has been recently published. Its intended audience is mainly student nurses and it covers most of the documents they need for their studies.

2 The authors of this research report are all affiliated with a university in the UK, and most of them have previously published in other international journals. The report was fairly recently published (2005) and its contents follow the typical layout of a research report. It presents evidence that shows the benefits and the shortcomings of post-partum smoking-cessation interventions based on the Transtheoretical Model (TTM).

3 Purdue University is a well-known and prestigious university in the USA. Its online writing lab has been created to help students improve their academic skills. The faculty in charge of developing the materials are all qualified and experienced teachers. The materials are quite varied and cover most aspects students may need for the development of their academic skills.

4 Spiegel's text is a classical reference in psychopharmacology. This is its fourth edition. Spiegel is a senior industrial pharmacologist and is affiliated with a university in Switzerland. The author's contributions are well known in the field.

Chapter 4

ACTIVITY 4.1

Experience	Description	Reflection
Discontinue breastfeeding	Visit to the client's house The client's house Client's anxiety and reasons for it What the student midwife did What the midwife did	Client's need for information to make informed decisions. Realizing the importance of consistent supervision and advice

ACTIVITY 4.2

In general this is a good conclusion. However, it could be improved if the writer made it more balanced by adding something about the other skills discussed in the introduction and the body of the reflective essay. Also, the conclusion would need to specify the course of action for the needs identified in the body paragraphs.

Chapter 5

ACTIVITY 5.1

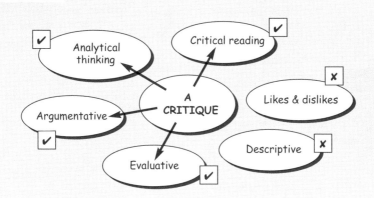

- Analytical thinking ✔
- Critical reading ✔
- Likes & dislikes ✘
- Argumentative ✔
- **A CRITIQUE**
- Evaluative ✔
- Descriptive ✘

ACTIVITY 5.3

① Identifies a well-defined problem

② States the focus clearly (issues)

③ Anchors topic in context

④ Signposts action by the care critique

In the UK there is wide recognition of the increasing number of patients with mental health problems who also misuse psychoactive substances. These substances range from alcohol, tranquillizers, barbiturates, heroin and stimulants such as amphetamines, cocaine and its derivatives, to cannabis and hallucinogens. Substances like these have an effect on the central nervous system in terms of altering moods, thought processes and behaviour. The combination of substance misuse and mental health problems is associated with a host of serious social, behavioural, psychological and physical problems, resulting in increased demands on mainstream services. As a result of their mental and health conditions, these dual-diagnosis patients face losing contact with friends, family and their homes. This critique will examine the care given to ten dual-diagnosis patients during the writer's clinical placement. More specifically, the critique will focus on the main factors that lead patients to lose contact with friends and family and the actions leading to the minimization of such loss.

(Markers: 3, 1, 2, 4)

ACTIVITY 5.4

This conclusion starts is a very effective way. It restates the identification of the main problem emerging from the care analysed and summarizes the major issues. However, in the last part it starts adding new issues that have not been mentioned before. This is exactly what conclusions should *not* do.

ACTIVITY 5.5

The recommendations made are appropriate to the topic examined. They have also indirectly revisited the weaknesses of the care critiqued, and made a point of discussing how to solve this problem.

Chapter 6

ACTIVITY 6.1

1 OP. It offers no support for the claims made.

2 FA. It uses references from the existing literature to support the claim made.

3 OP. It offers no support for the claims made.

4 OP. It offers no support for the claims made.

ACTIVITY 6.2

Topic: Risk assessment scales for preventing pressure ulcers	
Argument A (FOR): Using risk assessment scales (RAS)	**Argument: B (AGAINST): Scales have a major limitation**
Strengths	Weaknesses
• been developed since 1960s • variety of instruments • statistical comparison of different scales	• 'true' sensitivity of any RAS cannot be measured when preventive interventions are initiated.

ACTIVITY 6.3

1 *Many professionals:* Who? How many?

2 *Results of research in midwifery care are inconclusive:* What results? Of what previous research?

3 *It has, for example, been suggested:* By whom? When? Where?

4 *Health promotion programmes:* Examples at the national level? Examples at the local level?

References needed to be able to answer all these questions.

ACTIVITY 6.4

(1) Statement of the topic, (2) Argument or arguments that contradict the thesis, (3) Transitional marker showing a contradiction, (4) Statement of the thesis.

Text 1

The debate surrounding evidence-based practice and the implementation of research-based knowledge in practice is well rehearsed. Some of the key issues discussed have been perceived as barriers to the implementation of knowledge, with Funk *et al.* (1991) developing a 'barriers to research utilization' questionnaire that has been widely adopted in the National Health Service (Retsas 2000; Closs *et al.* 2000; Parahoo 2000) (1). However (3), these barriers have been mostly framed as individual responsibility – the lack of skill in research critique, the lack of interest in accessing the written knowledge base, the lack of compliance with the evidence (Kaluzny *et al.* 1995; French, 1996) (2). (Clarke & Wilcockson 2002, p. 397)
    No statement of thesis made (4).

Text 2

While (3) in recent years there has been an increase in the number of studies examining occupational stress among community mental health nurses (Harper & Minghella 1997; McLeod 1997; Coffey 1999; Drake & Brumblecombe 1999; Burnard *et al.* 2000) (1), the experiences of staff in acute inpatient settings, providing 24-hour care for people with serious mental illness, have received less attention (2). An investigation of acute mental health nursing commissioned for the United Kingdom's (UK) Department of Health (Higgins *et al.* 1997) has highlighted the need for further research in this area (4). (Jenkins & Elliott 2004, p. 623)

ACTIVITY 6.5

Version 2

It is possible, however, that the differences seen are not entirely explainable by disappointment with the care-giver assignment. Staniszewka and Ahmed (1999) point out that patients' expectations are influenced by their awareness of what they might realistically expect. Evaluation of a service is also influenced by beliefs about the duty the service owes the client and whether or not there were circumstances outside the service's control that affected the care (Williams *et al.* 1998). If expectations are a determinant of satisfaction with care, it is possible that there would have been less difference between the satisfaction scores of the two groups since women have different expectations for doctors than they do for midwives. (Harvey *et al.* 2002, p. 266)

Chapter 7

ACTIVITY 7.1

Patient's name	Mrs M	
Medical record number	ICD-9-CM 348.1	
Room number	231	
Date	18.07.10	
Problem	Description	Goal
Loss of self-image and self-esteem	Patient presents severe loss of self-image and self-esteem due to chemotherapy.	Will regain some self-image and self-esteem in 20 days.
Approach	Assessment	Review
Encourage patient to gradually return to normal activities.	Assessment in 21 days.	After first assessment.

ACTIVITY 7.2

Text 1 is part of the introduction of the report, and Text 2 is the abstract.

Chapter 8

ACTIVITY 8.1

Text 2 shows more variation. Not all its sentences start the same way and it shows a combination of short, simple and more complex sentences.

Nurses can work in many health-care settings, <u>which gives them</u> the opportunity to gain experience in all aspects of caring for clients and their families. Nurses can thus build their professional career in many different ways. <u>For instance, they</u> may choose to become clinical specialists or consultant nurses, or they can opt for managerial positions as a head of nursing services or supervisor of other nurses. <u>For the more academic-oriented ones</u>, there are also opportunities in education and research. <u>These are just a few</u> examples of the opportunities that nurses currently have to develop their professional interests.

ACTIVITY 8.2

<u>Cutting and repairing an episiotomy, and repairing vaginal/perineal lacerations</u> were each proposed and retained as basic skills. <u>Repairing a cervical laceration</u> was proposed and retained as an additional skill. <u>There</u> is considerable Grade I evidence that avoiding episiotomy enhances both short- and long-term perineal integrity, supporting the midwifery philosophy of non-intervention. <u>This evidence</u> is counter-balanced by other Grade I evidence that restricting the use of episiotomy increases the risk of anterior perineal trauma.

ACTIVITY 8.3

As pressure to control hospital costs has intensified, the need to deliver the best nursing care in the most economical way has grown. Internationally research reviews show the benefits of home care. <u>For example</u>, dialysis patients can be reunited with their families and hospital beds used only when really necessary. <u>In addition</u>, by reducing hospital stays, governments undoubtedly save thousands of dollars. <u>Nevertheless</u>, it is not possible for professionals and policy-makers to estimate the resource implications of in-home services in Hong Kong unless systematic research is undertaken. (Luk 2002, p. 269).

ACTIVITY 8.4

Text 1
This seems to indicate that to be effective smoking cessation intervention should consider both the foetus and the mother. **Summarize**

Text 2
To provide client-centred care, nurses should recognize culture-sensitive practices and their relation to social cultures. **Mark a transition**

ACTIVITY 8.5

Text 1
In contrast to this prevailing view of women as objects, many international leaders and agencies have taken action to promote women as persons with full human rights, beginning with the female child. (Thompson 2002, p. 189)

Text 2
Psychiatric and Social Work pre-admission assessment have long-standing histories as requirements of UK Mental Health Acts (1983). Pre-admission nursing assessment has no such obvious legal authority; however, the practice is commonplace for most, if not all, Medium and High Security Hospitals.

Despite the widespread nature of this practice, pre-admission nursing assessments have received little descriptive or research attention in forensic mental health. (Watt *et al*. 2003, p. 645)

Text 3
The women in the midwifery group were seen by an obstetrician during their initial visit to the midwives' clinic and at 36 weeks' gestation to confirm their low-risk status.

Apart from the two mandatory obstetrician visits, the midwives made autonomous decisions on the care they provided. They made referrals to, or consulted with, obstetricians and other health team members when the need arose. (Harvey *et al*. 2002, p. 262)

Chapter 9

ACTIVITY 9.1

Text 1
This text plagiarizes the original one by using practically the same ideas and words. Also, it claims that 'Several studies have suggested...' but it gives evidence of only two.

Text 2
This text correctly uses cites the information in the original text using different words. In other words, it doesn't plagiarize.

Text 3
This text not only plagiarizes the original one by using practically the same words, but also quotes the original texts incorrectly.

ACTIVITY 9.2

In general terms, it could be said that Text 2 presents a better version of a redefinition. However, it can also be said that there was actually no need to redefine Chlamydia in the first place.

ACTIVITY 9.3

Lifted version
A funded pilot programme in midwifery support in a community where this support was not available provided the authors an excellent opportunity to compare this service with that of existing maternity services for women at low obstetric risk. One of the major concerns in the region, probably as a result of not having this kind of care before, related to safety.

Improved version
Harvey *et al.* (2002) compare the quality of the service provided to low-risk women by existing maternity services and a new midwifery pilot programme. As midwifery services were not previously available, it was felt that the safety of the new practice should be given top priority.

ACTIVITY 9.4

Text A
The reported text is a good example of paraphrasing. It has kept the ideas in the original, but has changed most words and observed referencing rules.

Text B
This is a very poor example of paraphrasing. It is, in fact, an example of plagiarism. The reported text has not only used most of the words in the original text but it has changed some of the original ideas (e.g. patient values). It has also ignored referencing rules by lifting the last part of the original text and attributing it to Ingersoll.

ACTIVITY 9.5

To paraphrase you have to	✔	✘	?
1. Read the original and change a few words.		✘	
2. Read the original, underline main ideas and rewrite them in your own words.	✔		
3. Summarize the main ideas in your own words.	✔		
4. Summarize the original text, mostly using the same words.		✘	
5. Change some of the ideas in the original text, but use your own words.		✘	
6. Keep the ideas in the original text and express them in your own words.	✔		

To paraphrase you have to	✔
1. Read the original, keeping the same ideas in it but rewriting it using your own words.	✔
4. Summarize the original text, mostly using your own words.	✔
5. Keep the same ideas in the original text, but use your own words.	✔

Chapter 10

ACTIVITY 10.1

Text A: Anchoring the text in the field

Text B: Supporting ideas

Text C: Building an argument

ACTIVITY 10.2

Text 1: Critical stance

Text 2: Scaffolding

ACTIVITY 10.3

Reference 1 (Philips P. & Joanne Labrow 1998) has included the authors' name initial and name. This is incorrect, as in-text references should only show surname(s).

Reference 2 (Rassool 2001, pp. 110) has used the abbreviated form for pages (pp.) rather than the one for page (p.).

Reference 3 (www.mind.org.uk) has incorrectly included the webpage rather than the name of the page (Mind, National Association for Mental Health, 2006).

ACTIVITY 10.4

Courtenay, M. 2002. Movement and mobility in R. Hogston & P.M. Simpson (Eds.): *Foundations of nursing practice*, 262–85. Basingstoke: Palgrave.

Year of publication should be given in brackets. The same holds for page numbers which should be preceded by pp.

Johnson, T. and W. Taylor. (2005). *Skills for midwifery practice*. Second edn. London: Churchill Livingstone.

Jasper, M. (2003). *Beginning reflective practice: Foundations in nursing and health care*. Cheltenham: Nelson Thornes.

These references are not in alphabetical order.

Savage, T.A. (2005). How do we handle conflicts with parents over unsafe oral feedings? *Rehabilitation Nursing*, 30 (pp. 7–8).

Place of publication and publisher should be given at the end of the reference.

ACTIVITY 10.5

These pairs of sentences illustrate some of the functions of reporting verbs:

- In 1.1 by using the reporting verb 'provide', the writer is **merely saying** what the study he/she is referring to **did** ('provides an analysis of...'). In 1.2, on the other hand, by using the reporting verb 'claim', the writer is **discussing other people's views or beliefs** in relation to the study being reported.
- In 2.1 the writer uses 'find' **to describe the results of the study** s/he is reporting on. In contrast, in 2.2 the writer chooses 'criticize' to indicate what **the authors he/she is referring to believe**. This is **further emphasized** by the use of the adverb 'strongly'.
- In 3.1 the use of the reporting verb 'repeat' **merely indicates** that such an idea appears in the text more than once, whereas in 3.2 the use of 'reiterate' (repeat for emphasis) indicates **the author's views** on the importance of such an idea.

ACTIVITY 10.6

1 = C

2 = B

3 = A

4 = C

5 = A

ACTIVITY 10.7

Examples	Function	Tense	Reason for choice of tense
1. Crowe *et al.* (2016) <u>have argued</u> that improving the care of older people who suffer from multimorbidity is a considerable challenge for most health-care systems worldwide.	To discuss other people's ideas, views or beliefs	'have argued': present perfect	Introducing a topic or idea, with a focus on the ideas rather than the time
2. In their 2009 study, they <u>tested</u> the internal consistency and reliability of their data-collection instruments on a group of 46 subjects.	To describe previous research activities or methods	'tested': simple past	Describing processes and procedures
3. Based on the results of their study, they <u>concluded</u> that improved self-efficacy of birthing women could help them deal with previous psychological trauma of giving birth and lower their psychological and physiological stress.	To report on a previous experiment or study	'concluded': simple past	Making reference to the results of the experiment or study
4. Shaw (2015) <u>has pointed out</u> that caring support from early stages of pregnancy in midwifery services is the most effective way of providing women with a positive birth experience.	To discuss other people's ideas, views or beliefs	'has pointed out': present perfect	Introducing a point of view, with a focus on the ideas rather than the time
5. His study <u>demonstrated</u> statistically significant effect sizes and improvements in fitness and physical activity of the subjects in the experimental group.	To report on a previous experiment or study	'demonstrated': simple past	Making reference to the results of the experiment or study
6. Using purposive sampling techniques, 25 research participants <u>were chosen</u> from the list ensuring diversity to take part in the focus groups.	To describe previous research activities or methods	'were chosen': simple past (passive voice)	Describing processes and procedures

7. Thomson and Downe (2010) highlight that a strong connection between the birthing woman and the midwife is a simple but effective way to achieve a positive birth experience.	To discuss other people's ideas, views or beliefs	'highlight', 'is': simple present	Emphasizing what is being reported
8. Allgood and Kvalsund (2005) have indicated that predictability is linked to a more mature phase in the relationship where mutual dependence is developed.	To report on a previous experiment or study	'have indicated': present perfect, 'is linked': simple present (passive voice)	Emphasizing what is being reported

References

Aston, J., E. Shi, H. Bullôt, R. Galway & J. Crisp. (2006). Quantitative evaluation of regular morning meetings aimed at improving work practices associated with effective interdisciplinary communication. *International Journal of Nursing Practice*, 12, 57–63.

Clarke, C.L. & J. Wilcockson. (2002). Seeing need and developing care: Exploring knowledge for and from practice. *International Journal of Nursing Studies*, 39, 397–406.

Cottrell, S. (2017). *Critical thinking skills: Developing effective analysis and argument*. 3rd edn. London: Palgrave.

Creedy, D.K., J. Horsfall & J. Gamble. (2002). Developing critical appraisal skills using a review of the evidence for postpartum debriefing. *Australian Journal of Midwifery*, 15, 3–9.

Davis, E. (2004). *Heart & hands: A midwife's guide to pregnancy and birth*. 4th edn. Berkeley, CA: Celestial Arts.

Driscoll, J.J. (1994). Reflective practice for practise – A framework of structured reflection for clinical areas. *Senior Nurse*, 14, 47–50.

Durgahee, T. (1996). Promoting reflection in post-graduate nursing: A theoretical model. *Nurse Education Today*, 16, 419–26.

Gibbs, G. (1988) *Learning by doing: A guide to teaching and learning methods*. Further Education Unit. Oxford: Oxford Polytechnic.

Harvey, S., D. Rach, M.C. Stainton, J. Jarrell & R. Brant. (2002). Evaluation of satisfaction with midwifery care. *Midwifery*, 18, 260–67.

Health Encyclopaedia, NHS Direct. Available at www.nhsdirect.nhs.uk/en/CheckSymptoms. Last accessed on 23 January 2014. NHS Direct was dissolved in March 2014 so this website is no longer available.

Hjelm, K., P. Nyberg & J. Apelqvist. (2002). Gender influences beliefs about health and illness in diabetic subjects with severe foot lesions. *Journal of Advanced Nursing*, 40(6), 673–84.

Jenkins, R. & P. Elliott. (2004). Stressors, burnout and social support: Nurses in acute mental health settings. *Journal of Advanced Nursing*, 48, 622–31.

Johns, C. (2004). *Becoming a reflective practitioner*. Oxford: Blackwell.

King, J.F., V. Flenady & L. Murray. (2002). Prophylactic antibiotics for inhibiting preterm labour with intact membranes. *Cochrane Database of Systematic Review*, 4, CD000246.

Kravits, K., R. McAllister-Black, M. Grant & C. Kirk. (2010). Self-care strategies for nurses: A psycho-educational intervention for stress reduction and the prevention of burnout. *Applied Nursing Research*, 23, 130–38.

Kritsotakis, G., M. Psarrou, M. Vassilaki, Z. Androulaki & A.E. Phi-Lalithis. (2016). Gender differences in the prevalence and clustering of multiple health risk behaviours in young adults. *Journal of Advanced Nursing*, 72(9), 2098–113.

Luk, Suet-Ching W. (2002). The home care experience as perceived by the caregivers of Chinese dialysis patients. *International Journal of Nursing Studies*, 39, 269–77.

Maughan, K., B. Heyman & M. Matthews. (2002). In the shadow of risk. How men cope with a partner's gynaecological cancer. *International Journal of Nursing Studies*, 39, 27–34.

McDaid, C., S. Hartley, A.M. Bagnall, G. Ritchie, K. Light & R. Riemsma. (2005). Systematic review of effectiveness of different treatments for childhood retinoblastoma. *Health Technological Assessment*, 9(1), 1–145.

Oshima, A. & A. Hogue. (1998). *Writing academic English*. 3rd edn. London: Longman.

Papanikolaou, P., M. Clark & P.A. Lynea. (2002). Improving the accuracy of pressure ulcer risk calculators: Some preliminary evidence. *International Journal of Nursing Studies*, 39, 187–94.

Popil, I. (2011). Promotion of critical thinking by using case studies as teaching method. *Nurse Education Today*, 31(2), 204–07.

Purdue University Online Writing Lab. Available at http://owl.english.purdue.edu. Last accessed on 23 March 2018.

Reeves, S., J. Goldman, J. Gilbert, J. Tepper, I. Silver, E. Suter, & M. Zwarenstein. (2010). A scoping review to improve conceptual clarity of interprofessional interventions. *Journal of Interprofessional Care*, 25(3), 167–74.

Rolfe, G., D. Freshwater & M. Jasper. (2001). *Critical reflection for nurses and the caring professions: A user's guide*. Basingstoke: Palgrave.

Schon, D.A. 1987. *Educating the reflective practitioner: Towards a new design for teaching and learning in the professions*. San Francisco, CA: Jossey-Bass.

Swales, J. & C.B. Feak. (1994). *Academic writing for graduate students*. Ann Arbor, MI: University of Michigan Press.

Thompson, J.E. (2002). Midwives and human rights: Dream or reality? *Midwifery*, 18, 188–92.

Van Manen, M. (1977). Linking ways of knowing to ways of being practical. *Curriculum Inquiry*, 6, 205–28.

Watt, A., B. Topping-Morris, T. Mason & P. Rogers. (2003). Pre-admission nursing assessment in a Welsh medium secure unit (1991–2000): Part 1 – An analysis of practice and cost. *International Journal of Nursing Studies*, 40, 645–55.

What is Plagiarism, Available at www.plagiarism.org/search?q=Plagiarism. Last accessed on 23 March 2018.

Widmark, C., C. Tishelman & B. Ahlberg. 2002. A study of Swedish midwives' encounters with infibulated African women in Sweden. *Midwifery*, 18, 113–25.

Index